Dogmatic Diets

How Fad Diets Influence The Way We Live, Eat, And Discuss Nutrition.

James E. Clark

Dogmatic Diets: **How fad diets influence the way we live, eat, and discuss nutrition**.
Copyright © 2024, James Clark.

Dogmatic Diets: **How fad diets influence the way we live, eat, and discuss nutrition**.
ISBN: 9798328136471

Other publications are available at:
https://sites.google.com/view/scientifichealthpublications/home
https://rss.com/podcasts/scientific-health-education-human-performance/
https://www.youtube.com/@Scientific.Health.Education
https://jeclark.substack.com

Dedicated to all of my students.
The former, the current,
and the future ones.

Dogmatic Diets

How fad diets influence the way we live, eat, and discuss nutrition.

Table of Contents

Preface.
Welcome to this book.

To begin, thanks for opening the cover of this book and for your willingness to read my thoughts about diets and the influence that diets have on the opinions that we try to spread to others. Influences that shape our ideals and tenets for how to eat and how to live in an attempt to be healthy, wealthy, and wise. Or at least healthy. Ideals that we use to build our lifestyles around, becoming the foundational blocks for why we eat the way we eat, why we exercise the way we exercise, why we live the way we live... to some it takes the shape of our worldview much in the same way that religions shape our world view.

While it can be beneficial for the person, it can also be the fundamental reason why having a non-combative and intelligent conversation about diet and lifestyle tends to be problematic. Since too many of us become entrenched in our own point of view and neglect the advice of the ancient Greek philosophers, who spoke of wisdom as being able to speak to both sides of an argument and instead hold fast to the opinion that their diet and dietary belief system are the best way to diet without accepting that they might be wrong.

A problem that becomes exaggerated by a desire to oversimplify how the body works and a poor understanding of what happens in our body from the food that we eat. Poor understanding about how the body works is further complicated by bad logical arguments and the use of bias in rationalization for why some diets are better than other...issues that are seen across the litany of publications that we see on the topic. And tend to form many of the ill-advised statements, misinformation, and disinformation that are both the cause of and cure for the plague of non-communicable diseases of the 20th and 21st centuries. Biases that impact the validity of arguments seen in some very popular books, websites, social media broadcasts, and dietary programs that we buy into as being a way that I can finally reach the body image I want and have the health that I have long desired to have. Problems that I hope to address as we progress through the discussions contained in the pages that follow.

Dogmatic Diets stem from my attempt to address these problems and misunderstandings that are realized when I lecture on the topic of diet, nutrition, and metabolism to health science students. Lectures where students are taken aback by the simple statement that "Calories can't be burned" because it challenges one of the most common misunderstandings about metabolism and the human body. As we are reminded through every advertisement, every social media post, and every conversation we might have about trying to lose weight, we have to eat fewer Calories than we "burn" doing exercise. Also, it is important to note that the book and diets being discussed here are not focused on the ideal of weight loss, even though that is what we tend to focus on when we talk about diets. It really stems from the wonderful conversations that I have had with students throughout my career teaching future healthcare professionals and some contentious conversations that I have had with teaching colleagues at a few colleges in the United States.

Discussion where colleagues have voiced their desire to teach nutrition courses, so that they can teach about their diet. Without realizing the impact that projecting a specific lifestyle has on what students will project to others without realizing the mimicking effect that they are performing. In conversations with colleagues, I began to see the biases and logical fallacies that have clouded their judgments and blinded them from viewing anything else as having validity. A blindness to biases that all-to-often have crept into the larger discussions that we have around diets and dietary practices. Practices that I have come to notice take on the hint of being religious in the implications and insinuations for why someone should follow the diet. Where it feels like we are being preached to instead having an open dialogue with an exchange of opinions and ideas.

Thus, the purpose here is to not covert you. It is an attempt to inform you and let you know a little about what can happen inside your body and to your health should you choose a diet to use. In attempting to address the problems and answer these questions, I am not going to simply provice a summary of what is believed. Or, as some have done in the past, insinuate that believing a specific diet is fundamentally good or bad. Doing either would simply propagate the issues that I am attempting to address. Instead, the discussion will flow using the following template:

- Summary of the foundation of the dietary practice
- The central ideas and tenets of the diet, including implied benefits
- The benefits and risks of following dietary practices based on human physiology and the evidence we know that has come from experimentation
- What can we say about the diet? The pros and the cons
- A take home message about how you can apply the diet into your life without having it become a dogmatic way to live.

But, before we get ahead of ourselves, it is important to first address some of the concepts that we do a horrible job with... educating everyone on the basic scientific concepts and terms.

All the big words...
a quick foray into scientific terms and concepts

"You keep using that word,
but I don't think it means what you think it means"
--Inigo Montoya, **The Princess Bride**

Before we jump into why we are here, it is important that we get some of the boring stuff out of the way first. The ability to understand the truth about what diets can do for your health, or if claims about different diets are valid, is to approach them scientifically. Most of us are not too thrilled about that idea, because a lot of us have had bad experiences with science class in the past or had a boring teacher droll on using big words that we could never quite understand. Well, to help this aspect of our discussion, I want to try to define a few key words and then discuss some of the issues that we see across the discussions we have about diets, nutrition, and how our body works.

Key terms to be aware of

One of the things that we are constantly doing in science is speaking in "big" words that can be confusing to someone who is not familiar with how scientists communicate or when scientists forget who we are communicating with... as Alan Alda famously quipped, "If I understood you, would I have this look on my face?" Which brings me to the opening of the book, providing some useful definitions for words that you will see throughout the discussion. While I have tried to simplify as much as possible, there are just some key terms that cannot be reworded to not be scientific. They are not being left in as a "Look how smart I am; my argument must be correct." Nor are they being left in as a way to make you feel like this book and the discussion about diets here are more correct than other books that have been printed on these topics. It is simply that the words are the words, and there is no way around not using them.

Without further ado, here are some key terms (in alphabetical order).

- **Acid:** a substance that reduces the pH of a solution
- **Acidosis:** a health condition where there are more acidic substances in the bloodstream than the body is able to remove
- **Anti-nutrient:** a substance that can be found in food we eat that interferes with the digestion, absorption, or use of a nutrient that is found in the food we eat or use in the body
- **Alkaline:** a substance that increases the pH of a solution
- **Alkalosis:** a health condition where there are more alkaline substances in the bloodstream than the body is able to remove
- **Bioavailable:** when a nutrient or chemical is able to be absorbed and used by a cell of the body. Relates to issues of deficiencies and anti-nutrients seen with some diets

- **Bliss and Bliss Point:** the feeling of joy that comes from eating food and is associated with desires for having more of that food
- **Calorie:** the amount of heat that is needed to raise 1 liter of water 1 centigrade, equivalent to 4.1868 Joules or 1.163 Watt*hours. Mistakenly discussed as something that can be burned by the body, but cannot as it is a measure of energy that we are losing from the reactions making up our metabolism
- **Concentration:** the reference given to the amount of the substance we are looking at in a solution based on the total amount of solution
- **Deficiency:** a state where there is a shortage of specific nutrients that comes from either not having it in the diet or not eating enough to offset the amount being used by the body, having another chemical interfering with its use
- **Disruptor:** a substance that will stop or slow metabolism or change metabolism that leads to health issues developing for the person. Normally described as a **metabolic disruptor** if the chemical impacts the metabolism of a cell or tissue only, or an **endocrine disruptor** if the chemical impacts how a specific hormone might function in the body.
- **Endocrine:** term that is used to cover chemicals that can tell cells of the body when changes in metabolism is required.
- **Excite or Excitation:** an increase in the responses and processes in the cell, tissue, or organs of the body based on need to maintain homeostasis
- **Feedback:** a processes of using messages between the cells, tissues, and organs of the body that either inhibits or excites responses that is used to maintain optimal performance and homeostasis
- **Feedback dysregulation:** state where a feedback is not correct that leads to disease, can be associated with metabolic disruptors, endocrine disruptors, or overfatness.
- **Homeostasis:** state of optimal performance where the cells, tissues, and organs of the body are able to perform as required. Directly relates to being healthy
- **Hypothesis:** explanation for why something happens based on currently understanding and knowledge
- **Inflammation:** responses in the body that changes metabolism associated with tissues being hurt or someone being sick or having a disease
- **Inhibit or Inhibition:** the reduction in responses or processes in the cell, tissue, or organs of the body necessary to maintain homeostasis

- **Macronutrient:** substances that are necessary in the diet in large amounts and are typically stored as the molecules used to build the tissues that make our body
- **Metabolism or Metabolic process:** the total of all chemical reactions and responses in the cells, tissues, and organs of the body that allows for optimal performance or are done an attempt to get back to optimal performance. This term gets confused with how much energy is being used but is not the same thing.
- **Metabolite:** the term given to any chemical or molecule that is used by the cells or tissues of the body during metabolism
- **Micronutrient:** substances that are essential to our body being able to perform optimally, but are not needed in large amounts
- **Nutrient:** any substance in our food that can be used by our body to maintain optimal conditions and performance
- **Overfat and Overfatness:** a health status that is associated with what people call obesity but can occur without diagnosis of obesity. Typically, a diseased health status that develops from disruption of metabolism and high amounts of inflammation.
- **Regulation:** control of the processes through feedback that either excites or inhibits metabolic processes throughout the body
- **Soluble:** ability for a substance to form into a solution with a liquid. Typically describe substances as being **"lipid soluble,"** or substance forming a solution in a fatty liquid or oil, or as being **"water soluble,"** or a substance that forms a solution with water.

Let's talk a little about science

Misconceptions about how we do science lead to the installation of a pseudoscientific approach. Pseudoscience allows for misinformation and disinformation to flourish in our discussions about diet, nutrition, and health.

How to tell if you are dealing with information based on science or pseudoscience?

The biggest way to tell the difference is based on what evidence is being accepted and the confidence that one has about something being proven true;

see table Words1. One of the easiest ways to differentiate is that pseudoscience tends to speak in definite absolutes of certainty, while science tends to speak in conditional terms of certainty. A difference that brings me to a confession about what science does, that almost everyone gets wrong... science is not done to **prove something to be true**.

Table Words1. Basic principles that can be used to show the differences that exist between science and pseudoscience.

Science	Pseudoscience
<ul><li>Tests hypothesis for truthfulness without preconceived notion for outcomes</li><li>Follows the evidence and changes opinions based on evidence to draw a conclusion</li><li>Makes tentative claims and conditional conclusions</li><li>Embraces criticism and corrective feedback regardless of where it comes from</li><li>Engages with peers and non-peers in the community to reach and explain a consensus</li><li>Follows a logical process of analysis that considers all points within an argument equally and without prejudice</li><li>Uses rigorous and reproducible method of investigation and analysis to draw a conclusion</li><li>Uses clear and precise terminology with operational definitions being provided when necessary</li></ul>	<ul><li>Sets out to prove a conclusion instead of testing a hypothesis</li><li>Hostile to criticism and corrective feedback</li><li>Grandiose claims and conclusions that may not be true based on empirical evidence</li><li>Ignores evidence that contradicts opinions and beliefs, while cherry-picking favorable evidence that supports opinions</li><li>Uses logical fallacies and inappropriate analysis as basis for rationales and justifications</li><li>Uses poorly constructed methodology that is not well defined, explained or reproducible</li><li>Disengages with community and peers in the research process when forming a consensus or opinion about a truth</li><li>Speaks in jargons, incorporating confusing and vague terminology</li></ul>

Instead, science is used to test the how, what, when, where, and why something occurred and then explain our results based on our current understanding about how our body works. Because our understanding of the evidence must be supported or refuted based on our current understanding, our ability to draw conclusions and make recommendations must also change as our knowledge of how the human body works changes. This also means that if someone is relying on one report, even if it happens to be the latest report, to justify their decision about a diet, it can lead us to think incorrectly about what that diet might do, or, more importantly, not do in our strive to be healthy.

When we examine why a diet might work, we tend to look for **cause-and-effect relationships**, even if we make one up using correlations between what we are seeing. To see if a cause-and-effect relationship exists, we must do so by following the scientific method and being logical in our thinking. Logical thought that will either be deductive, using what others have said and attempting to explain why something happened, or be inductive, using empirically collected results and fitting those results into the general rules about how our body functions to explain why something happened. Deductive reasoning will allow us to develop the hypothesis, our explanation about what we are seeing before doing an experiment, while inductive reasoning is going to be used to form our conclusion, how we can explain what we saw after performing the experiment.

To help in this process and keep us from falling to our biases, employing logical fallacies, or embedding pseudoscience into our arguments, here are some simple ideas to remember:

1. All explanations must be based on careful observations that come through testing a hypothesis that explains what we are questioning.
2. Any hypothesis has to have the possibility and probability of being disproven (evidence from observation does not support the hypothesis).
3. Conclusions cannot be based simply on one's opinion or beliefs about how the body works.
4. Any observations must be explained based on the principles of physiology that can be sensed and perceived in the same way by everyone, all the time.
5. That the best conclusion is the choice for explaining the phenomenon that has the greatest amount of factual support, is based on logical analysis, and makes the least number of assumptions to "best fit" all of the facts from the observations (Occam's Razor).
6. Scientific consensus is not democratically fair. There is no vote to say that something is true or not. The consensus is based on all of the available information, critically analyzed using a logical flow of thought

free from bias or logical fallacy, and it says what is true, even if it might challenge our preconceived notions

Limiting your bias and eliminating logical fallacies

When trying to understand how a diet might impact our body, we must use Occam's Razor and be very careful to limit assumptions we have to make in order to form our conclusions. The fewer assumptions, the more likely we are to be thinking correctly; sometimes this idea gets oversimplified to the simplest answer being the correct answer. At the same time, we must avoid biases or committing logical fallacies in forming our explanations. A few times throughout this book I will mention how bias and fallacies are impacting the validity of the claims that proponents of various diets are voicing, and to help understand why that might be taking place, it is important that we are all at least exposed to the most common biases and fallacies. Not only so that we know what needs to be avoided, but also what we can do to minimize our bias or reliance on logical fallacies when discussing diets with our friends, family, and anyone else that might come in earshot of such conversations.

What is bias?

Bias is a change in perspective about the truth that distorts results or leads to false conclusions. It can occur anytime you are gathering information about how the human body functions (including collecting evidence, performing analysis and interpretation, or discussing your conclusions about what was found). Being aware of bias is important. But understanding how bias exerts its effects is even more important for several reasons. Bias can exist in every discussion we have about diets and what they can do, is very difficult to eliminate, and adversely impacts the validity and reliability of your interpretations of findings.

Because of this, it's crucial for you to be aware of the potential types of bias, so you can minimize them. To help, let's look the most common biases that one might fall for:

- **Confirmation bias**: Bias results when we choose only the data that supports what I want to be true and ignore everything that might disagree with me. Most common of the biases and gets associated with a number of other biases, while being linked with *cherry-picking* or *the Texas sharpshooter logical fallacy*, and possibly the *moving the goalpost logical fallacy*
- **Observer bias:** Tendency to see what we expect to see or what we want to see. That is, we use our prejudice to examine and interpret any information or observations (whether consciously aware of the prejudice or not).
- **Outlier bias:** Bias that is caused by relying on data that greatly differs from the rest of the results and skews conclusions to the outlier and away from the importance of all other observations, leading to erroneous conclusions.
- **Analysis or Cognitive bias:** Bias in data analysis comes from reliance on subjectivities, implicit or overt motivations, to prove something to be **true**. Allows our prejudices about what we wanted to be **true** to cause us to overtly rely on unrepresentative data, or answers to leading questions, or a combination of the two when forming our conclusions. This generally goes unnoticed until a decision is challenged for be ng an erroneous conclusion about the validity of the results.
- **Faulty interpretation:** A form of confirmational bias where one approaches analysis of information in order to only justify a belief or opinion that focuses on a select portion of information that supports the point of view while ignoring the remainder of the data set as being faulty.
- **Anchor bias**: Bias that uses personal perspectives or anecdotes or a single data point to draw a conclusion about why something is occurring. The reason that these are not valid for developing a conclusion is that using anecdotes or a single point of observations falls prey to the logical fallacy of hasty generalizations, limiting the validity of the conclusion drawn from a single data point.
- **Performance or Actor bias:** Bias that occurs when applying outcomes to a treatment while knowing that participants knew they were being

treated. This is where if I am told a diet will have specific benefits, I am more aware of seeing those benefits or having physiological responses that mirror those benefits. Sometimes referred to as the placebo effect, but more often is an example of a Hawthorne effect, as we tend to unknowingly change our actions and then attribute benefits (or harms) to just coming from the diet and nothing else.

How would you limit or combat bias?

It is very difficult to eliminate bias; however, there are a few things that we can do to limit its effects on our thinking. The first thing to do when combating bias is to accept that we have biases. When you understand that you have a bias whenever viewing your evidence, you are less likely to function in a biased manner. Accepting that you need to let go of your biases means that you are able to go where the evidence takes you, not where you might want to take the evidence.

To help you meet this ideal, here are a few simple rules that I try to follow to limit my own bias:

1. When analyzing information, cognitively separate yourself from what you think the evidence might show.
2. Check for alternative explanations and consider whether there are other reasons why the responses are the responses. Ruling out or accounting for alternative explanations of your interpretation makes your argument more correct.
3. Review findings with others and ask them to review your conclusions to identify logical gaps or assumptions in your argument that need to be addressed or if your conclusions are sound and reasonable given your current knowledge base.
4. Use others to help with the analysis and interpretation to look for consistency between everyone, as it is more likely that there is some truth when there is agreement between various independent interpretations.
5. Remember that every response will always show regression to the mean. A term that tells us that if we see stories that show extreme responses in a few measurements over time or when given enough measurements the value on the measurements will tend to move closer to the center (the mean or average) of all the measurements

6. Look at the information critically and follow a logical process of thought that eliminates logical fallacies.

What are logical fallacies?

Using inferential thinking to formulate the explanation for both what happened and why it happened can be problematic if we are not careful in how we establish our rationales. In performing your logical thinking to infer the explanation, you are linking your observed experimental results with the principles of human physiology. This means you have to go back to what we already know about how the human body functions and then apply what the results say about this understanding. You have to do this by limiting your assumptions and following a logical process of thinking. The logical process means that if you commit a fallacy in your thinking, then the entirety of your interpretation becomes nullified. Here are the most common fallacies that are used in defense of our dietary choices that we need to be aware of:

- **Hasty Generalization:** This is a conclusion based on insufficient or biased evidence. In other words, you are rushing to a conclusion before you have all the relevant facts. Typically comes from the use of anecdotes or a single study. These are the "I did this, and it worked, so it must work for you too."
- **Post hoc ergo propter hoc/Because it happened last, it must be the cause:** This is a conclusion that assumes that if 'A' occurred after 'B,' then 'B' must have caused 'A.' Typically comes from the use of faulty cause-and-effect rationalization. These are the "I did this, it worked, so it must be because I did this." Without looking at all of the other things taking place (the Hawthorne effect).
- **Begging the Claim:** conclusion that is provided is proven as being validated within the claim of that very conclusion. Typically comes from stating the principle or law is the observation. These are the "Smith's law says this occurs and this occurred due to Smith's law..." where their responses being observed are not discussed or put in context of the law

- **Tautology/Petitio Principii/Circular Argument:** a restatement of the argument rather than actually proving it. Also called a tautological statement. Typically comes from making the clause (subject) of the statement the rationalization for the statement. These are the "I did something, and my heart rate changed because I did something."
- **False Dichotomy, False Dilemma, or the Either/Or argument:** a conclusion that oversimplifies the argument by attempting to make the complex too simple by "dumbing it down" too much. These are the statements of "the changes happened because of either this… or that… occurred" when there are hundreds of possible causes and rationales.
- **Ad populum/Bandwagon Appeal:** a conclusion that appeals to what most people, or a group of people, thinks in order to persuade one to think the same way without offering factual evidence to support claims as being true or not. Typically, it comes from an overreliance on popular opinion or misunderstanding of how scientific consensus are developed. These are the "people say…" or "I read online that…" statements.
- **Ignoratio Elenchi/Red Herring:** a diversionary tactic that avoids the key issues, often by avoiding opposing arguments rather than addressing them. Typically involved within the "hot button" issues of health science, where the key aspects are not addressed while opinions and not facts are overly expressed and relied upon. These are the "it has to be because we only see it in…" statements.
- **Straw Man:** oversimplifies an opponent's viewpoint to make it a false argument and then attacks that false argument. See with the "hot button" issues of health science where a false impression is given to what is being stated while not offering justifications for one's own argument. These are the "the only reason to make that choice is because you are in favor of all similar choices…" statements.
- **Argumentum ad ignorantiam/Appeal to ignorance:** offers no proof of anything except that you don't know something. Typically involved with conclusions where limited understanding exists on the key aspects that might explain the responses seen. These are the "we don't know much about…" statements.

- **Slippery slope:** conclusion that offers the argument that the outcome will likely lead to further outcomes that do not logically flow because there is no evidence. Typically seen with the "hot button" issues of health science, where oversimplifying the counterarguments presents an inaccurate set of potential cause-and-effects that cannot be supported based on what is known. These are the "if we make that choice, it will cause all of this to occur…" statements.
- **Tu Quoque:** conclusion does not provide an argument but distracts from the argument due to a position that the opposing view only occurs because of a hypocrisy in the opposing viewpoint. Typically involves flipping the argument back to the person making the argument, which most often revolves around openness to lifestyle treatments for health issues. These are the "I'll do this, yet you do this, too…" statements.
- **Ambiguity/Equivocation:** a statement is offered to confuse or mislead by requiring one outcome to be the same as another. Typically involves flipping the meaning of words by removing the context of the word in the discipline. These are the "it's just a theory" statements without recognizing that in scientific communication, a theory is the rationale for why laws are true versus the idea of a theory being a "guess" as used outside of science.
- **Non sequitur:** a conclusion does **not** follow logically from what preceded it. Typically involves connecting two things occurring that have nothing to do with each other. These are the "this occurred… then that occurred… the occurrence of this must be with that…" statements, such as "When I am around cake, I have to eat all of the cake; therefore, I must be addicted to cake."
- **Argumentum ad verecundiam/Appeal to Authority:** Conclusion that is justified because of citation of an experiment that agrees with the conclusion. Typically involves the overreliance on one to two "experts" that justify the position that one is taking. These are the "research says…" statements that do not reflect on how the observations relate to those statements.
- **Non causa pro causa/Causal Fallacy:** stipulates that the cause is based on and around unproven relationships. Typically involves poor analysis in the cause-and-effect relationship or using correlation as a means to justify causation. These are the statements that do not reflect the timing of an event or the impact of other factors in the outcome.

- **Cherry-picking and Bull's Eye or Texas Sharpshooter Effect:** forming a conclusion by using only selected evidence to be used in the argument to support the point of view or forming the correctness of the argument based on a heavily-biased selection of materials that only agree with personal point of view. Typically, is used in cognitive and confirmation biases.
- **Moving the Goalpost Effect:** constantly changing how much evidence needs to be produced to provide enough support to allow for the correctness of the challenging point of view. These are the "well, what about this..." statements, where there is never enough evidence for the person questioning to accept a different point of view.

With some background information taken care of, let's start our discussion about diets by first addressing how we like to think and talk about diet and the lifestyle that comes from our diets.

Diets, are they really our new religion?

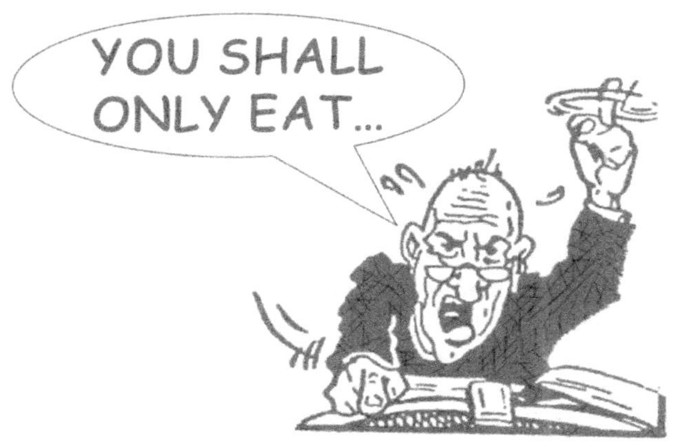

Religious practices often entail following distinct and sometimes restrictive eating habits. So much so that the idea that eating and diet are something beholden to religion is not a new idea and is commonly accepted as a cornerstone of many cultural aspects of our health, a concept that many have previously written about. As many religious leaders both implicitly and overtly offer dietary recommendations through religious laws that followers are expected to use, that should be seen as providing nutritional advice. Advice that does impact the nutritional status of the followers and is based on how nutrition impacts metabolism and the health of these believers. These dietary practices come in many forms; the most of us are aware of foods being **kosher** (Jewish dietary laws), **halal** (Islamic dietary laws), and **ahimsa** (Hindu dietary laws); and that religions like Mormonism (Latter Day Saints), Seventh Day Adventists, and Buddhism offer advice to restrict certain types of foods and food products from one's diet.

Yet, at the same time, we have come to understand that we live in a secular world. A secular world with many different religions, different cultures, and different dietary practices. Something that has been recognized, at least tangentially, for centuries. And have, once again at least tangentially, recognized that our diet will impact how well we are able to live …

> *"Tell me what you eat, and I will tell you who you are."*
> *—Jean Anthelme Brillat-Savarin*

To wit, we currently like to think about food and diets as ***you are what you eat***. Yet the ways that we eat, even within many of the diverse food cultures, have shown to be as highly variable as everything else within the faddishness of our current secular culture. Faddishness of lifestyles can really be the only explanation for the billions of dollars spent each year on unproven elixirs and remedies for any one of the noncommunicable diseases that plague us, or to generate the aesthetic body image that would ease our psyche and make us feel complete. We freely consume untested or quality-controlled herbs and supplements. Faddishness has extended to diets and dietary trends where we consume all-meat diets, no-meat diets, grapefruit diets, and caveman diets, and we switch from killer butter to margarine and back to butter. Faddishness can take on the ideals of religious dietary practices, which can truly impact our overall health.

A variability that falls back on the way that our body uses the nutrients that we get from our food. Which means that to understand diet and nutrition, we must also understand metabolism and the basics of chemical reactions taking place inside every cell of our body every second of every day. Whenever I teach the topic of metabolism, it always starts from the premise that metabolism is meaningless without acknowledging the concepts of diet and nutrition. An approach to the topic based on the premise that I have regarding diets as being the plan used to meet my nutritional needs required for my metabolism always introduces the diet portion of the lecture with the following slide:

DIET...A FOUR-Letter Word?

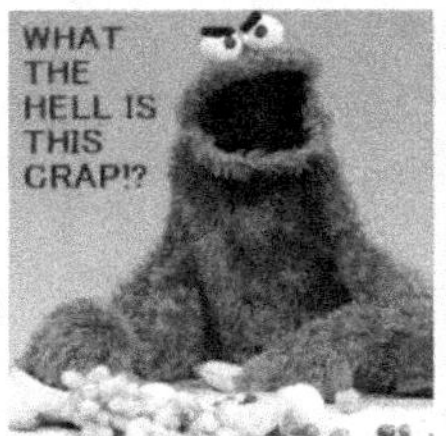

A slide meant to counter how we tend to think of diets as what is being restricted and not what is consumed-- as something that is to be avoided or something that comes inherently with punishments attached to the foocs we like to eat, *a moment on the lips... a lifetime on the hips...*

A thought about diets that have grown from over the decades of teaching metabolism this way, continually refining the discussion with students, and realizing that students approach diets from a philosophical perspective more than a scientific discussion. Making me wonder if we have flipped the narrative about diets and religions, questioning not if religions determine our diet but **if our diet is forming a religion.**

Well, let's look at the hallmarks of religions and see if they fit into how we all can approach diets. In which I will try to not veer into the oncoming train of the proselytizing aspect of dietary lifestyles. But then again, that seems to be a given to most diets and is the reason we tell ourselves why we need to avoid talking about our lunches with **Keto Kerry** and **Vegan Vance** at all costs...

How can we determine if the diet is a nutrition plan or a religion?

Based on the idea that diets are meant to ensure that you get all the food that you need to meet your body's needs for a day, it seems like a ***no-brainer*** in the discussion here. Meaning that you're going to say, "of course diet is a nutrition plan." Something that is readily recognizable by glancing through any nutrition textbook or discussing diets with a registered dietician. But what about the second half of the question, something that can become evident by glancing through any of the diet books that weigh down the shelves at your local bookstore?

To answer this part of the question, it is first important to define what we mean by religion. Here I turn to Merriam-Webster and see that **religion *is a set of organized beliefs, practices, and systems that most often relate to the belief and worship of a controlling force***.

Since religion tends to take on its definition as a social contract, i.e., a culture, it is important to expand this definition into a purpose for the organized beliefs and practices in one's everyday life. Where I will summarize this purpose to be a source of comfort and guidance that forms the basis for beliefs and behavior while providing one with a sense of community and connections to a set of traditions that can be relied upon as a reason for one's lifestyle. A culture that stems from the practices and traditions of the family and one's home while binding them into their interactions with everyone and everything within the greater society of people.

But how does this idea of religion equate to the ideas about diet? Well... if we were to take steps of exploration about religion that many religions hope we would take during their maturation process, the selection of one's religion can come down to three key features:

#1: A community that you connect with
#2: Utilizes practices that purport wellness as its primary benefit
#3: Provides material that inspires you to continue its practices

Based on these three key features of religion, it's not a stretch to see how we embed religious dogmatic practices into our approach to diets. Regardless of those diets being the latest fad or a well-studied and entrenched part of medical interventions.

Community you connect with

This is where we can view many of the dietary restrictions that world religions offer as the simplest means for a diet forming a religion (or a religion forming a diet). When we select a popular diet, we get a sense of aligning ourselves with a way of eating that promotes a sense of belonging to something larger than ourselves. A community of others that are acting and behaving as I do, a network of support that I might need should I cheat or falter in my ability to maintain my diet. That is, by changing the way I eat, I essentially become a member of a club I didn't know about.

Where my group of dietary friends and family allows for social meeting places (i.e., restaurants, community cookouts, etc.) that give me a sense of belonging. Places that should I follow a different diet, I would no longer be accepted at. A place and community that offers me a sense of belonging, a phenomenon that applies to many churchgoers from the least to the most devout of the congregation.

Practices that purport wellness

While this is not an exhaustive list, a lot of the dietary practices that we get exposed to purport an ability to:

- lose body fat
- avoid or remove toxins
- reduce inflammation
- reduce diabetes
- improve memory and mental clarity
- reduce cancer
- reduce heart disease
- improve bone health and muscle strength

Wellness is coming from the diet, but only if we would follow their guidelines and practices. With the premise that if we stray from dietary practice, you do not get the benefits of wellness.

Inspire you to continue its practices

This is where the relationship between diet and religion seems to lock arms and why the **Paleo Paul**, **Keto Kendra**, or **Raw-Food Randy** are always talking about their diets... try to convince you to join their group of like-minded eaters. Rely on their anecdotes, their personal stories of success, to win us over to their dietary practice.

A practice that we see across the gamut of the diet culture books that weigh down the shelves at the bookstores around the world, fill our internet searches, and endlessly fill our social media feeds.

Diet zealotry... a way to live?

Food and diet zealotry is nothing new. Many of the foods that we take for granted come from food zealotry, from soft drinks to breakfast cereals. The ability to be agnostic in the face of ever more religiosity taking hold of diet and nutrition means needing to understand the scientific consensus about the benefits and harms that can arise from strict adherence to dietary practices.

So, what are some of the diets that will be discussed? Well, the popular ones that tend to have the greatest amount of religious fervor behind them, such as:

- Atkins Style
- Bland
- Carnivore
- Clear Liquid
- Detox
- Diabetic (Low Glycemic Load)
- Full Liquid
- Full Plate
- High Fiber Diet
- Ketogenic
- Low-Carbohydrate Style
- Low-Fat
- Low-Potassium
- Low-Residual Fiber
- Low-Sodium (DASH)
- Mediterranean
- Mindful Eating
- Paleolithic
- Plant-Rich (Vegan)
- Raw-Food
- Zone (Proportionality) Diet

Where the intention is to examine the pros and the cons, the scientific evidence to support or refute the use of these various diets. A presentation of the ideals and core concepts that hopefully will provide you with a knowledge base to accept or reject dietary practices without intentionally converting anyone to do so dogmatically.

Calories go in...
Calories go out...

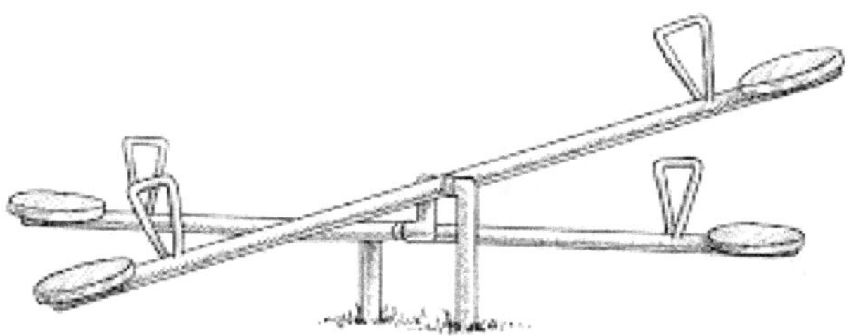

I think it is best to start where almost all discussions about diet tend to start, the idea of the Calorie and Caloric Balance.

Okay, a quick question... when I ask you about nutrition, how quickly do you immediately start thinking about the number of Calories you are eating?

If you answered, "Yes!" That's great. If you answered, "Well, no, I think about what I am not supposed to eat." That's great, too. The way in which diets and nutrition are sold is based on these two ideas; what not to eat and how many Calories are in the foods we are eating.

It is a normal thought to think about food based on Calories and our "2000 Calorie per day" limit. But here is another question we need to ponder. A two-part question that is more important than the opening question. What the heck is a Calorie and why do we care about Calories?

To start the answer, we need to address one of the finer points regarding Calories that almost all of us get wrong at some point of the discussion. Calories are unable to provide your body weight and definitely cannot be burned-- because they are not a structural physical thing. They are a unit of heat; specifically, they are the amount of heat necessary to raise 1 kilogram (kg) or 1 liter (L) of water 1 degree Centigrade.

From this point, we need to reflect in our discussion that a Calorie is going to be the energy (heat) released from the chemical reactions taking place in our cells that allow us to live, to exercise, and to do activities we enjoy doing. This idea means that we might expend Calories in activity from our metabolism, but how does that relate to our discussion here? Through the concept of our metabolic rate, the idea has led to the popular labeling of foods with Caloric content and percentages based on 2,000 Calories per day. That 2,000 Calories is the indicated metabolic rate, with the faulty presumption that everyone has the same metabolic rate.

Caloric Balance and BMR Calculations

While we commonly discuss metabolic rate based on energy expenditure, it is important to remember that metabolic rate is simply the measure of the amount of metabolism completed per unit time and not necessarily the amount of energy being expended. Yet we still reference metabolic rates based on the daily expenditure (Cal/day). A value that more honestly should be called our total energy expenditure (TEE) and not our metabolic rate. Where metabolic rates are the amount of metabolism being completed to maintain and grow the tissues of the body, the TEE is telling us how much energy is being expended at rest (REE), during activity and exercise (AEE), or from digesting the foods we are eating (TEF). Simplified to the equation:

$$TEE = REE + AEE + TEF$$

Even with all of the technology we wear, it is still incredibly difficult to obtain a true measure of energetic cost for any activity or from all of the metabolism we do in a day. This means that to determine our energy requirements for a day, we estimate our needs, an estimation that has become oversimplified to be represented by 2,000 Calories per day on the food labels that we see. Estimations that we can all determine are through a variety of mathematical equations that provide us with an indicated basal metabolic rate (BMR) that is really just our estimated TEE. Even with a host of equations available, the Harris-Benedict and Katch-McArdle equations tend to be the most popular for determining our estimated BMR, Table Calories1.

One of the keys that we take away from all of the estimation equations is that there is a slew of factors that can and do impact our estimated BMR or TEE. Of these factors, we must divide them into the modifiable (e.g., those factors that we have influence over: level and duration of habitual activity, health status, body mass, and composition, societal attitudes on diet) and non-modifiable (e.g., factors that we cannot control: age, gender, ethnicity, height). Take a minute to use the equations to estimate your BMR and note its relationship with the 2,000 Calories that we see printed everywhere. It is important that a caveat is raised here.

Table Calories1. Equations used for the estimation of basal metabolic rates (BMR) for adults.

Equation Name	Mathematic Equation	Factors
Cole (Normal weight)	Male: $e^{-0.16310.00255 \cdot A+0.4721 \cdot BM+0.2952 \cdot H}$ Female: $e^{-0.1934-0.00199 \cdot A+0.4764 \cdot BM+0.0194 \cdot H}$	BM=Body Mass (kg) H= Height (cm) A=Age (years, to closest year)
Cole (Overweight/ Obese)	Male: $e^{-0.2630-0.00277 \cdot A+0.4877 \cdot BM+0.3367 \cdot H}$ Female: $e^{-0.0713-0.00209 \cdot A+0.4075 \cdot BM+0.3540 \cdot H}$	BM=Body Mass (kg) H= Height (cm) A=Age (years, to closest year)
Harris-Benedict (pounds and inches)	Female: $((4.36 \cdot BM+4.3 \cdot H-4.7 \cdot A)+665) \cdot ACF$ Male: $((6.23 \cdot BM+12.7 \cdot H-6.8 \cdot A)+66) \cdot ACF$	BM=Body Mass (pounds) H=Height (inches) A=Age (years, to closest year) ACF= activity conversion factor (energy expenditure beyond resting metabolism) 1.2 (only activities of daily living) 1.4 (light activity 3-4 days/week) 1.6 (moderate activity 3-4 days/week or light activity ≥5 days/week) 1.8 (high activity 3-4 days/week or moderate activity ≥5 days/week)
Harris-Benedict (metric)	Female: $((9.6 \cdot BM+1.8 \cdot H-4.7 \cdot A)+665) \cdot ACF$ Male: $((13.7 \cdot BM+5 \cdot H-6.8 \cdot A)+66) \cdot ACF$	BM=Body Mass (kg) H=Height (cm) A=Age (years, to closest year) ACF: same as above
Henry/Oxford	18-to-30-year-old: Females: $0.0546 \cdot BM+2.33$ Males: $0.0669 \cdot BM+2.28$ 30-to-60-year-old: Females: $0.0407 \cdot BM+2.90$ Males: $0.0592 \cdot BM+2.48$	BM= Body Mass (kg)

Katch-McArdle	9.6•FFM+370	FFM=Fat-Free Body Mass (pounds)
Mifflin-St Jeor	Female: 10•BM+6.35•H-5•A-161 Male: 10•BM+6.35•H-5•A+5	BM=Body Mass (kg) H=Height (cm) A=Age (years, to closest year)
Schofield	18-to-30-year-old: Females: 0.062•BM+2.036 Males: 0.063•BM+2.896 30-to-60-year-old: Females: 0.034•BM+3.538 Males: 0.048•BM+3.653	BM= Body Mass (kg)

Let's try to figure out a BMR for a fictional person using the Harris-Benedict equation for a man that is 30 years old, stands 5 ft 9 in (or 69 inches), and weighs 170 lbs.

$$\text{Male BMR} = ((13.7 \cdot BM + 5 \cdot H - 6.8 \cdot A) + 66) \cdot ACF$$

$$BMR = (13.7 \cdot 170 + 5 \cdot 69 - 6.8 \cdot 30) + 66$$

$$BMR = (2{,}329 + 345 - 204) + 66$$

$$BMR = 2470 + 66 = 2536 \text{ Calories/day}$$

He works out 3 times a week at moderate intensity, which gives an ACF of 1.6 that we will multiply our BMR by. Meaning that we have an additional 60% above just resting requirements that need to be accounted for:

$$BMR = 2536 \cdot 1.6 = 4058 \text{ Calories/day}$$

Based on this example, if our guy were to eat based on the 2,000 Calories/day he would be under-consuming almost 2,060 Calories/day.

Now, try it for yourself:

Man: 13.7 x _______________ (weight)= _____________________________

+ 5 x ___________(height in inches)= ___________

- 6.8 x ___________(age in years)= ___________

= _______________________________ + 66 x _______________ (ACF factor)

= _______________________________

Woman: 4.36 x _____________ (weight)= ___________________________

+ 4.3 x __________(height in inches)= ___________

- 4.7 x _____________(age in years)= ___________

= ________________________________ + 665 x _______________ (ACF factor)

= ________________________________

What is important to recognize before we move on is that the estimated value determined from many of these equations may not accurately establish a true set point for the person. As most regression equations being used were developed based on white male college-aged populations that might not reflect the entire population or were established from groups that were weight-stable and healthy. Meaning that for women, minorities, under-represented populations, or those changing lifestyles to lose or gain weight, using many of the established equations may not provide an accurate representation of estimated energetic needs. Meaning that 2,000 Calories might be the requirement for one person, but not necessary for me or anyone else because of how the variety of factors involved will interact with each other.

The influence of modifiable factors leads to two big myths about Calories and BMR being ingrained in the discussion about Calories and nutrition and diet and health. The first, which actually leads to the second, is that there are "fast metabolism" and "slow metabolism" people. While metabolic rates will fluctuate, the changes in BMR from day to day, stress to stress, can speed up or slow down our metabolism; this does not mean that we have "fast" or "slow" metabolism. Stemming from this misconception is another, more problematic thought, that increasing fat-free mass (i.e., skeletal muscle) has an impact to elevate BMR while increasing fat mass depresses BMR. However, it appears that this thought is not supported by research, as fat mass (i.e., adipose tissue) is a very metabolically active tissue and not simply an inert tissue storing lipids for later use as a fuel source. An idea that we have previously thought to be true and in some subgroups of society still holds on to as being factual. A combination of ideas that lead to problematic recommendations when we start looking at breaking down diet into a balance.

A balance of intake and expenditure. A balance that we tend to think of as a teeter-totter or a seesaw, where if intake is greater than expense I gain, or if I flip that balance to favor expense over intake I lose. And the gain and loss are always referenced as body weight.

Calorie Balance or Nutrient Balance—what's more important?

In order to understand the discussion of the balance, it is important to do a quick dive into some science quickly. Components of our diet typically are broken into two classifications, macronutrients and micronutrients, or "macros" and "micros" of our diet. Interestingly, the way we talk about these components based on a balance point varies wildly from each other. Where "micros" are typically discussed based on nutrient balance, where we see values of grams per day (g/day) or grams per pound (g/lbs). Yet, when we discuss Caloric balance, we are looking at the relationship of Calories coming predominantly from the "macros" of our diet (e.g., carbohydrates, lipids, proteins) relative to how we use these nutrients to meet the fuel demands for generating energy for the body. Based on this balance, we typically assign 4 Calories per gram to our protein and carbohydrate macronutrients and 9 Calories per gram to our lipid (fat) macronutrients. Where we are essentially looking at the amount of potential energy that is contained within the molecules, the food that we eat is meant to replace energy stores used during the day.

Even though the conversation about balance and body weight (or composition) both within and outside of healthcare and fitness focuses on the concept of the Caloric balance, where the central tenet focuses on the idea that consumption of more Calories than expended in activities throughout the day would lead to weight gain, while the opposite is associated with weight loss. There is actually limited evidence for establishing a negative balance (more expending than intaking) as being effective for long-term weight loss, weight maintenance, or body compositional changes.

A finding that seems perplexing, as it appears to be that Caloric balances are used out of apparent simplicity and popular applications. Rationale has several logical flaws that hamper its overall justification for altering or maintaining body mass. The first and most important challenge to this fallacious rationale for using a Caloric balance is the rhetorical question that should be constantly raised: ***how much does a Calorie weigh?***

Nothing. Calories are massless units of heat, and as such, Calories cannot contribute to weight.

As such, it might be time to question the validity of Caloric balance as an explanation for weight gain, weight loss, or body compositional changes that are being attempted through dietary modification. Not only because of possible flaws in the estimation of energetic demand but more importantly, what the Caloric balance does not consider about our diet. That food is consumed and used for other metabolic processes beyond those associated with energy. There is growing evidence that we should address our "macro" needs similar to how we address our "micro" needs for nutrients. That is consuming given amounts of each "macro" based on a relative amount (grams) for our body mass (lbs or kg). This idea of nutrient density for "macros" necessary to maintain tissues and normal metabolic function means that per day we should consume:

- carbohydrates at a range of 2.5-3.5 g/kg or 1.13-1.7 g/lbs. (on the low end) up to 5-10 g/kg or 2.25-4.5 g/lbs. (on the high end) with 120-130 g/day

For our man that we used to calculate BMR, that means needing to consume between 192 and 765 g/day.

- proteins at a range of 0.8-2.7 g/kg or 0.36-1.0 g/lbs. (with 6 g/day of Creatine, and maximum of 12-15 g/day branch-chained amino acids)

For our example, that means needing to consume between 62 and 170 g/day.

- lipids a range of 0.8-1.1 g/kg or 0.36-1.0 g/lbs. 2-3 g/day Omega-3 and 12-17 g/day Omega-6 (maintaining ratio of 1:6 Omega-3 to Omega-6), with trans fats capped at 2 g/day and saturated fats capped at 20 g/day.

For our example, that means needing to consume between 62 and 170 g/day.

Go ahead, take a second and look at your ranges now:

- Carbohydrates: _____________ and _______________ g/day

- Protein: _____________ and _______________ g/day

- Lipids: _____________ and _______________ g/day

While a lot of diets will use the Calories/day values and the balance points within their tenets, one set of dogmatic diets is entirely reliant on it, the proportionality diets.

Proportionality diets

The idea and concept about proportionality diets stem from addressing a wider question about dieting. Is there some secret formula I can follow to ensure I get a 'balanced' diet in each meal?

As we might be able to surmise from every food commercial we see stating that their meal is part of a balanced diet, there really is not some secret formula to ensure that you have a "balanced" diet, a ratio for macronutrients in your diet based on the factors that influence need. Yet, many who follow the guides of the proportionality diets will speculate that having a 'balanced' diet can be achieved based on using a ratio of Calorie balance being 40-60% from carbohydrates, 20-30% from protein, and 20-30% from fats. Further differentiation of the proportionality diets from the other dogmatic dietary practices stipulates that to achieve 'balance' in our diet, we determine proportions and ratios within any meal based on the following questions:

- What is my nutrient and Caloric balance point?
- How many meals will I be eating throughout the day?
- What is the quality of the nutrients in the foods? Am I consuming complete proteins? Which is important; if you only consume plant sources of proteins, then you need to look at ways to get amino acids that may be missing some of these essential amino acids.
- What type of foods do I have allergies to or select to not consume?
- Am I getting enough fiber? The fiber is typically consumed in the form of leafy vegetables and whole grain cereals (oats, wheat).

What is key in proportional diets versus other dogmatic dietary practices is that addressing these questions comes not from necessarily indicating "good food" or "bad food" within the dietary practices. Instead, the focus is on the balances within the diet. The Caloric balance. The nutrient balance. The balances that provide our guidelines for servings and serving sizes of the foods and food groups that make up our diet.

Meaning that when discussing diets, it is no longer discussing what is being cut from the foods that we eat, but on the concentration of the "macros" that we consume on a daily basis. Where the primary discussion of proportionality diets is based on the foods we eat is essentially based on the amount of potential energy that is contained within the food that we eat to replace energy being used during the day. A proportionality of each "macro" is based on the contribution that each has to the Caloric balance point relative to BMR that we follow. Within proportionality diets, we see a variety of dogmatic systems that are practiced, from the popular **The Zone Diet** to the dietary practices preached by governmental organizations (e.g., MyPlate from USDA, EatWell Plate NHS (UK)) or public health advocates (e.g., Harvard School of Public Health's Healthy Eating Plate).

Food Pyramids, MyPlate and Food Groups:

The general idea of a proportional diet is to present simplified nutritional guidelines. The initial guides developed in the early 20th century that became solidified by the 1970s as the now-famous "food pyramids" with the four major food groups that we are familiar with:

- Milk and dairy products
- Fruits and vegetables
- Meat and meat substitutes
- Bread and cereals (grains)
- Fats and Oils

The original food pyramid and revised MyPyramid that gave way to the MyPlate for developing proportions of food in each meal or total servings in a day.

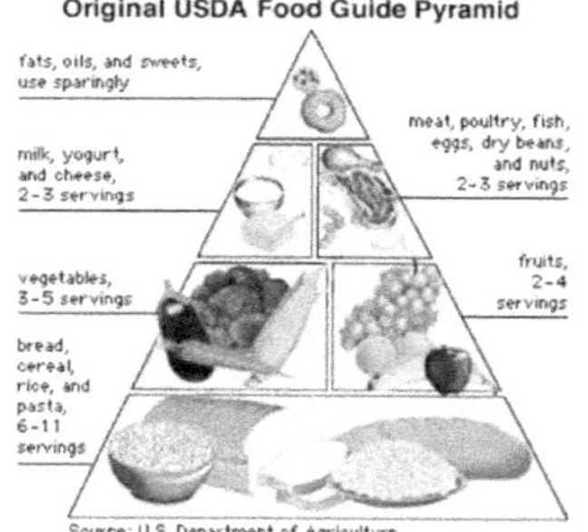

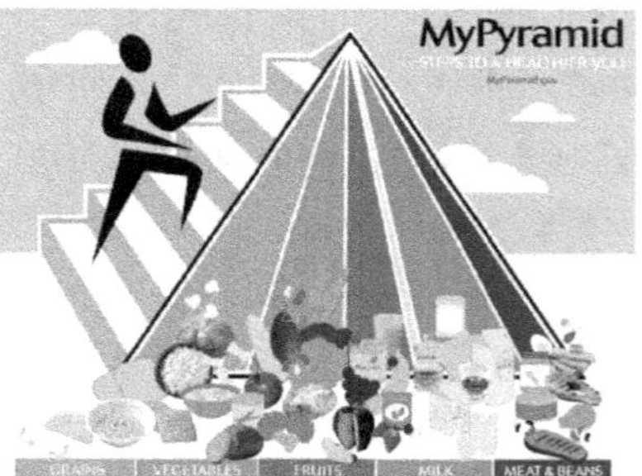

The general idea within the pyramid was to examine servings of the food groups that you eat, more than a discussion of serving sizes, nutrients, or Calories that might come from each serving. The pyramid was based on a majority of the servings coming from cereals or grains (6-11 servings), fruits (2-4 servings) and vegetables (3-5 servings), with fewer servings coming from dairy (2-3 servings), meat or meat substitutes (2-3 servings), and sparing use of oils, fats, and processed sugary foods.

This pyramidal model underwent revision to include physical activity in the late 1990s and early 2000s along with the introduction of personalized guidelines for food that increased the variety and proportional breakdown within the food groups. With the current version ditching the pyramid for the plate image in an attempt to better show the proportional relationship between the food groups. Imagery that focused on a secondary goal of this form of proportional diet, controlling overeating through teaching portion control within individual meals. The new imagery, while showing variance, typically indicated a defined proportion of meals being made of "grains," "vegetables," "fruits," and "proteins," smaller portions of a meal coming from "fats or oils," "added sugars," and "dairy."

MyPlate and the Healthy Eating plate that can be used as a guide for developing proportion of each meal.

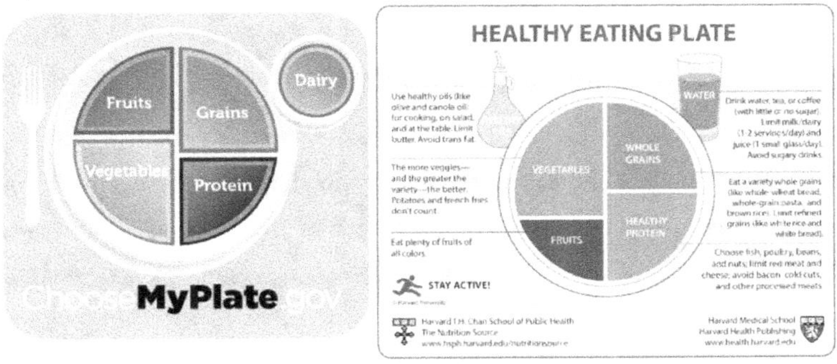

The general idea being that using a plate image would make it easier to observe portions of the food groups and use some degree of "common sense" when measuring amounts of food groups to eat. There was also the added benefit of using imagery as a way to help reduce salt (sodium) and sugar being consumed while giving greater freedom in choice for protein or grain sources. These early movements and the imagery that stemmed from them were not related to nutrient needs and balance or even the Calories and Caloric balance concepts that are the governing principles of proportionality diets that we see today. Instead, it was meant to teach portion size and ensure that a variety of foods were being consumed in a population that was becoming reliant on mass-produced and processed foods in their diet.

The Zone Diet and other Calorie-proportional diets

In the 1990s a secondary look at proportional diets hit the market with Barry Sears publishing his book **The Zone Diet**. The idea of the zone diet was to focus not specifically on the food pyramids and food groups, but to break the foods being eaten throughout the day into a relative proportion to each other based on the following ratio: 40% of Calories coming from carbohydrates, 30% of Calories coming from protein, and 30% of Calories coming from lipids (fats and oils). Within the implementation of the Zone Diet there are two general premises that need to be followed.

- Premise 1: the proportion of macronutrients in each meal is broken up into the ratio of: 40% Carbs:30% Fat:30% Protein.
- Premise 2: eat low glycemic fruits and vegetables in the carbohydrate portion of the diet.

The proponents of the diet stipulate that by following the two premises, you are able to reduce inflammation that comes from the diet and reverse chronic inflammation linked to metabolic issues (i.e., metabolic syndrome).

To successfully use the breakdown offered from **The Zone Diet,** we would first take the Caloric balance point that we might have for the day and then break that into Caloric balance point for each meal by dividing total Calories by the number of meals you eat. Then break our foods into carbohydrates, proteins, and lipids based on the 40%, 30%, 30% for each, respectively, and then convert that energy into the amount of food by the conversion factor of 4 Calories per gram of carbohydrate or protein and 9 Calories per gram of lipid. This means that we need to do several mathematical calculations for each meal that we are having each day. Here's an example using 2,000 Calories/day eating either 4-meals (equal Calories) or 3-meals (equal Calories):

2000 Calories/day ÷ 4 meals/day = 500 Calories/meal

OR

2000 Calories/day ÷ 3 meals/day = 667 Calories/meal

Carbohydrates

= 0.40 x 500 Calories/meal

= 200 Calories of Carbohydrates/meal ÷ 4 Calories/g Carbohydrates

= 50 g Carbohydrates per meal

OR

= 0.40 x 667 Calories/meal

= 267 Calories of Carbohydrates/meal ÷ 4 Calories/g Carbohydrates

= 66.75 g Carbohydrates per meal

Protein

= 0.30 x 500 Calories/meal

= 150 Calories of Protein/meal ÷ 4 Calories/g Protein

= 37.5 g Protein per meal

OR

= 0.30 x 667 Calories/meal

= 200 Calories of Protein/meal ÷ 4 Calories/g Protein

= 50 g Protein per meal

Lipids or Fats

= 0.30 x 500 Calories/meal

= 150 Calories of Fat (Lipid) /meal ÷ 9 Calories/g of Fat (Lipid)

= 16.67 g Fat (Lipid) per meal

OR

= 0.30 x 667 Calories/meal

= 200 Calories of Carbohydrates/meal ÷ 4 Calories/g Carbohydrates

= 22.22 g Fat (Lipid) per meal

Breaking these macronutrients further, **The Zone Diet** proponents stipulate that by controlling fats being consumed and increasing protein consumption along with focusing on carbohydrates coming from higher fiber fruits and vegetables, you are able to control inflammation and insulin resistance. Eliminate foods that are believed to prevent the optimal functioning and health of the body.

Within these recommendations, we are given that protein sources should come from what has been identified as "low-fat" meats or "lean proteins" like chicken and turkey breast, lean cuts of pork and lamb, fish, egg whites, vegetarian protein sources, and low-fat dairy (cottage cheese, yogurt) and avoid protein sources that might be seen as "fatty meats" like processed meats, bacon, sausages, whole eggs (including yolks), fatty red meat, hard cheeses, or full-fat dairy. While lipid (fat) sources should come from what are identified as "healthy" or "good" fats, like olives and olive oil, canola oil, olives, nuts and nut butters, avocado. Avoiding "unhealthy" or "bad" fats, like trans-fats, hydrogenated vegetable oils, lard, and animal fat. With carbohydrates coming from fruits and vegetable sources such as spinach, kale, peppers, lettuces, broccoli, cabbage, apples, melons, oranges, grapefruits, stone fruits (peaches, apricots), while eliminating or minimizing sugary beverages (juices, sodas) or low-fiber starchy carbohydrates like potatoes, processed grains (bread, pasta, cookies, crackers), rice, bananas, corn, mango, kiwi, or papaya.

Along with **The Zone Diet**, there are a number of advocated proportional diets that have been offered from medical and health associations, the most prominent coming from the American Heart Association (AHA), which offered a similar breakdown as Barry Sears. The AHA's proportional (see *I Need a Remedy...*) diet changes the Zone breakdown to use 50-60% of Calories coming from carbohydrates, 20-30% of Calories from proteins, and at most 25% of calories coming from fats, with less than 7% coming from saturated fats.

Refinement of the AHA version of the proportionality diet combined the ideals of the food pyramid's servings with the Caloric breakdown of the "macros," leading to recommendations of 5-10 servings of fruits and vegetables, use of whole grains and products made up mostly of whole grains, "healthy sources" of protein, minimal processed foods, and no added sugars or salts to food. With the focus of diet to move toward mostly plants and nuts or lower-fat dairy and animal proteins. The ideal that the proponents of the AHA diet offer is that lower fat and sugar and by limiting animal or saturated fat in particular reduces cholesterol levels in the blood, inflammation in the arteries, and thus would possibly allow for better heart health. While reducing salt intake helps reduce fluid volume in the body, it would reduce blood pressure and improve heart health. More on these ideas when we discuss the "DASH" diet.

Along with **The Zone Diet** and the diets from the AHA and other medical organizations, the general premise for a lot of the mass-marketed diets we see is based on proportionality and Caloric balance (see *I am one with my food…*). These include dietary programs from companies like NOOM, Jenny Craig, Weight Watchers, and SlimFast. Regardless of which mass-marketed program is being selected, the general premise is to follow a diet that reduces Caloric intake in total while shifting proportional Caloric intake away from carbohydrates (especially refined sugar carbohydrates) with a small increase in protein intake. The goal for all of the mass-marketed diets here is to induce weight loss independent of any changes in overall health or performance.

Nutrient balance and planning your diet

While we discuss the Caloric balance quite often and use it in the development of proportions in diets and even to serve as the foundation for the food pyramid/MyPlate, nutrient balance should be seen as more important for health and metabolism than the energy balance component to diet. It is this balance that we can see as being part of the focus of servings and serving sizes promoted by the pyramids and plates, along with the idea that guidelines can be used to develop an individually tailored plan that will meet metabolic demands. A concept based on the ideal that eating correctly is essential for good health and optimal performance, that stipulates you can only use the fuels and molecules in metabolism that are available, and the availability directly impacts metabolism and performance through influencing muscle strength and endurance, metabolic flexibility, cardiovascular endurance, immune response to stress, and neurological and cognitive function. These demands allow for the establishment of guidelines required for "macros" (carbohydrates, proteins, and lipids) and "micros" (vitamins, metabolites, and minerals) to provide the amount needed per day or relative to body mass versus by a percentage of total caloric intake for a day; see table Calories2. Where missing nutrient balance requirements lead to nutrient deficits will be discussed as we move through the various dogmatic diets in this book.

Macronutrients or the "Macros" of the diet

Carbohydrates have gotten a bad reputation, mainly around topics related to overfatness and metabolic syndrome, with people constantly discussing sugar spikes and insulin spikes as the rationale for avoiding carbohydrates. While insulin can spike with meals (it rises simply because we eat regardless of how much sugar is in what we are eating), the spiking that everyone is concerned about will only happen when there is a consumption of glucose greater than about 1.2 grams per kilogram (0.6 grams per pound) per hour within the meal. Meaning that a 100-pound person would need to consume over 60 grams (14.33 teaspoons) of sugar in 1 hour to trigger the insulin spike that we hear should be feared. What is even more important to know about carbohydrates for your nutrient balance is that they are essential for metabolic functions of very important tissues of the body (i.e., nervous cells, immune cells, skeletal muscle). So important that we need a minimum of 120-130 grams/day just for normal neuron functions. Additionally, it is important to also consume the complex carbohydrate known as fiber somewhere in the neighborhood of 30-50 grams of fiber per day. While fiber is not going to directly impact the function of tissues of the body, its presence in our intestines is essential for digestive functions and the health of the microbiome found there.

Table Calories2. Recommended values of macronutrient intake based on proportion of Calories/day, relative to one's body mass, or suggested daily intake.

Macro	Percent of Calories/day	Relative to body mass	Other suggested daily intake values
Carbohydrate	40-60%	Low-end: 2.5-3.5 g/kg or 1.13-1.69 g/lbs High-end: 5.0-10.0 g/kg or 2.27-4.54 g/lbs	Minimum Carbohydrate: 120-130 g/day Fiber: 30-50 g/day
Protein	20-30%	Normal: 0.8-2.2 g/kg or 0.36-1.0 g/lbs Weight loss or Old-Age: 1.85-2.25 g/kg or 0.84-1.02 g/lbs Exercise: 1.2-2.5 g/kg or 0.54-1.54 g/lbs	Branched-Chain Amino Acids: 6-20 g/day Isoleucine, Leucine, Valine Creatine: 3-6 g/day Essential Amino Acids: Arginine, Histidine, Isoleucine, Leucine, Lysine, Methionine, Phenylalanine, Threonine, Tryptophan, Valine
Lipid (Fats)	20-30% Saturated Fat ≤7%	0.8-1.0 g/kg or 0.36-0.54 g/lbs	Saturated fat: Maximum: 20 g/day Trans fat: Maximum: 2 g/day Omega-3: ALA: 2 g/day EPA and DHA: 1-2 g/day Omega-6: 12-17 g/day

For carbohydrates, we can state that we should consume along a continuum of 2.5-3.5 gram per kilogram of body mass (1.13-1.59 gram per pound) on the low end up to 5.0-10.0 gram per kilogram (per pound 2.27-4 54 gram per pound) the high end. To evaluate your balance point for carbohydrates, we calculate your carbohydrate load or the total carbohydrates that have been consumed each day minus the total amount of fiber being consumed. Understanding carbohydrate load is important, but there are secondary aspects of consuming carbohydrates that need to be understood. The type of carbohydrate and the metabolic responses seen in the body after eating these carbohydrates. A rationale that is behind the movement to limit the amount of "added sugar" found in our diet, so we are careful not to over-consume fructose. While we hear a lot about needing to monitor glucose and glucose levels in our body, fructose is a sugar that is known to actually change how cells use carbohydrates, promote food cravings, and increase lipid production. Actions that fructose will cause independent of any hormone (i.e., Insulin) spikes, and can lead to addictive eating and fat accumulation when fructose is in excess.

The other aspect of carbohydrate load that needs to be considered is the level of activity and possible desire to change body composition. If you are extremely active in endurance exercise, you should consume a carbohydrate drink solution at a rate of 0.8-1.0 grams per kilogram (0.36-0.54 grams per pound) of body mass per hour for restoring glycogen depleted from exercise. At the same time, we also know from studies on the low-carbohydrate diets that a consumption rate of 10-50 grams per day and 45-110 grams per day are safe and optimal for weight loss and weight maintaining, respectively.

Protein in the diet has become all the rage recently, and for good reason, as proteins have a valuable place in our metabolism. When looking at how much protein we need, the protein balance is a little more complex than we see for determining how much carbohydrate is need. More complex because we not only need to make sure we have enough protein but also have to look at the amino acids that are making up the proteins. In terms of consuming protein, there are a lot of different types and ways that you can get protein in your diet.

When we discuss types of proteins, it is generally based on the chemical structure of the amino acids within the protein or based on the quality of protein. Quality of protein is related to having a protein source that provides "complete" proteins, sources that provide all of the essential amino acids of the approximately 21 amino acids needed to make every protein that your body needs and other amino acids needed for metabolic functions. Of these amino acids, we have to consume several in our diet as they are deemed **essentials** because the body is unable to produce them (i.e., histidine, isoleucine, leucine, lysine, threonine, tryptophan, and valine) or we cannot produce enough to match the use of them in our normal metabolic processes (i.e., arginine, methionine, and phenylalanine). Along with needing complete proteins, the protein sources should also be able to provide the 6-20 grams of branched-chain amino acids and 6 grams of creatine that are necessary each day.

To make sure that we get enough protein, we have a general recommendation for protein to a range of about 0.8-2.2 grams per kilogram (0.36-1 grams per pound) of body mass, depending on age, attempting to lose weight, and how physically active you are. This range changes to 1.2-2.5 grams per kilogram (0.54-1.14 grams per pound) of body mass for those who are highly active, recovering from being ill, or trying to lose weight by following a lower Calorie diet. For those that are trying to exercise to gain muscle, you will need to increase your overall protein intake toward the higher end of the range, closer to the 2.5 grams per kilogram or 1.14 grams per pound, but there is really no logical reason to go beyond that upper end of the range, even if we hear a lot of talk that more protein means more muscle growth. From the evidence that we have, there is no true "additional benefit" obtained in either gaining or maintaining lean body mass in excess of 2.5 grams per kilogram (1.14 grams per pound) of body mass accompanying exercise. When we do see additive benefit going beyond the upper limit for protein, it is generally associated with low-intensity resistance exercise, when doing endurance exercise, or when exercise is used in combination with diet to lose weight. This reason for the additive effect in these conditions and not when lifting heavy weights is that the additional protein limits the breakdown of lean body mass by controlling cortisol that would break down protein either during the exercise or in response to fasting. Meaning that repair of the muscle occurs at a less negative (less breakdown) allowing for a better response rather than more protein itself causing the growth to occur.

For those who are older or are dieting to lose weight, excessive loss of lean body mass can become a problem due to cortisol and other hormones changing metabolism throughout the body. For these individuals, additional protein consumption can actually maintain lean body mass, even without exercising. With the greatest benefit at a consumption between 1.85-2.25 gram per kilogram (0.84-1.02 gram per pound) of body mass.

Of importance here is to remember that without reaching the minimal level of protein required in a day, the body will have a reduced ability to repair cells and tissues from the damage that simply living might cause. Signs that we can see when minimums are not being met include, but are not limited to, poor hair and nail growth, poor maintenance of lean body mass, loss of muscle and bone leading to reduced strength, and possible osteoporotic change in the bone. One group that becomes at risk for having protein deficiencies is elderly individuals, which is why this population will generally be advised, based on overall health status, to have a protein intake at the higher end of the range and closer to those that are dieting to lose weight.

Lipids (fats) consumption based on nutrient balance, like carbohydrates, have been susceptible to a bit of misinformation about the need within the diet. Just like proteins, we have to be careful when talking about fats, as the type of fat will determine the use of the fat and the impact that it has on overall health. In which there are fats deemed saturated fats, and then there are fats deemed unsaturated fats. Where saturated fats are typically seen as being "bad" dietary fats but are essential for metabolic process and unsaturated fats are typically seen as being "good" dietary fats. The unsaturated fats fall into two categories: the monounsaturated fats (MUFA) and polyunsaturated fats (PUFA). Additionally, you need to ensure that you are consuming appropriate levels of the unsaturated fats, the omega-6 and omega-3 fatty acids. These fats are commonly referred to as "heart healthy" and "brain healthy" fats, based on changes in liver and immune cell metabolism that limit circulating levels of "bad" cholesterol molecules (LDL) and inflammation impacting the body. Changes that limit the risk of vascular inflammation and development of atherosclerosis. Another name given to the omega-3 fatty acids is "essential" fatty acids, including three specific fats: alpha-linolenic acid (ALA), eicosapentaenoic acid (EPA) and docosahexaenoic acid (DHA).

While general guidelines for fats consumption are typically based on percentages of total Calories each day, we can provide a recommendation similar to carbohydrates and proteins with a range of 0.8-1.0 grams per kilogram (0.36-0.45 grams per pound) of body mass. This range is further broken down to the types of fats (saturated, unsaturated, trans fats) with a stipulated maximum of approximately 20 grams per day of saturated fat and 2 grams per day for trans fat. With evidence supporting that greater than 2 grams of transfats per day, regardless of the origin of the fat, can have metabolic-disrupting effect leading to inflammation and possible onset of non-communicable diseases (i.e., metabolic syndrome, cardiovascular disease, cancer), and based on dietary practice and overall lifestyle, excessive saturated fat intake increases the likelihood of heart disease. While one should consume approximately 3 grams per day of omega-3 (ALA, EPA, DHA) and 12-17 grams per day of omega-6, with a recognized ratio that one should consume about 1 gram of omega-3 fatty acid for every 4-6 grams of omega-6 fatty acid. The consumption of the omega-3 and omega-6 fatty acids in this ratio has been shown to have a protective effect against non-communicable diseases as well as being required for the production of the fats used to build the cell membranes in our body and produce a number of immune cell hormones necessary to regulate inflammation. When the ratio between omega-3 and omega-6 fatty acids is disrupted, especially when omega-6 fatty acids are being overconsumed, there is evidence to show increased inflammation and a reduced level of protection against non-communicable diseases. Interesting, even if the ratio of omega-3 to omega-6 fatty acids is met, we can see similar issues of increased inflammation and reduced protective effects when we have a dietary restrictions limiting EPA and DHA from our diet.

Micronutrients, or "Micros" of the diet

The designation of micronutrient is not one of lesser value but of lower required amounts when compared to the macronutrients that we have in our diet. When looking at micronutrients, we are generally talking about **vitamins, provitamins, coenzyme factors, or minerals (electrolytes)** that we need to eat in order to stay healthy. Micronutrients are atoms and molecules that are directly involved with our body's ability to perform metabolism, build tissues, and respond to disruptions in our health but are required in far lower total amounts each day relative to the macronutrients in our diet.

The recommendations are typically given based on the total amount that we need per day instead of based on one's body mass or as a percentage of Calories of food per day; table Calories3. Recommendations for a lot of the micronutrients are made due to effects that might occur because of deficits in specific vitamins or minerals impacting metabolism. In fact, a lot of the dogmas that we encounter have the potential to lead to deficits in some of the micronutrients. Risks that we have known for a long time that led to the fortification of many processed foods with vitamins and minerals to ensure that everyone is meeting their daily requirements, especially for B vitamins, vitamin D, Iron and Calcium. Fortification has gotten a bad reputation within some social media circles, but all fortification does is ensure that micronutrients that might be extracted during the processing of foods are added back into the final product. Thus, fortification can help prevent diseases like pellagra, scurvy, bone loss, excess fatigue, and cognitive malaise, anemia.

At the same time, it can lead to micronutrient toxicity due to overconsumption of foods recognized to have a high density of that specific nutrient. An issue that leads to a secondary recommendation for micronutrients is ensuring you are not overconsuming the vitamin or mineral. One mineral that is typically overconsumed is sodium, especially with the increased consumption of prepared foods and "sports drinks" or "electrolyte drinks" on a daily basis. There has also been an increase in the consumption of antioxidant vitamins (vitamin D, vitamin C) that, even though they have benefits within recommended ranges, can lead to oxidative stresses for cells when consumed in excess.

Table Calories3. Recommended intake for micronutrients of vitamins and minerals for average adults.

Fat Soluble Vitamin	Needed Amounts per day	Maximum Level per day	Water Soluble Vitamin	Needed Amounts (mg/day)	Maximum Level (mg/day)
A	900 mg	3000 mg	B_1	1-2	N/A
D	15-20 mg	50 mg	B_2	1-2	N/A
E	12-15 mg	1000 mg	B_3	14-16	35
K	90-120 mg	N/A	B_5	5	N/A
			B_6	1-2	100
			B_7	30	N/A
			B_9	400	1000
			B_{12}	2.5	N/A
			C	75-90	N/A

Mineral	Needed Amounts per day	Known Maximum Level per day	Mineral	Needed Amounts per day	Known Maximum Level per day
Calcium	1-1.2 g	2.5 g	Magnesium	270-350 mg	0.32-4.25 g
Chlorine	2-2.5 g	3.1 g	Manganese	1.8-2.3 mg	11 mg
Chromium	50-200 µg	1000 µg	Phosphorus	700 mg	4.0 g
Copper	900 µg	10,000 µg	Potassium	1.6-3.5 g	4.2 g
Florine	3-4 µg	10 µg	Sodium	0.5-2.3 g	4.0 g
Iodine	1.2-1.5 mg	6 mg	Sulfur	1.1-2 g	3 g
Iron	8-18 mg	45 mg	Zinc	8-11 mg	40 mg

What can we say about the Caloric and nutrient balance and proportional diets?

The general guidelines for most diets and dietary practices will stem from the idea of Calories and nutrients and the need to establish or maintain some sort of balance between what is being eaten versus what is being used on a daily basis. From this idea, we get general recommendations for how much of the macronutrients (carbohydrates, lipids (fats), or proteins) that are needed in a day either from the total Calories that each offers or based on necessity for metabolism based on relative body mass.

Pros:

- Offers general nutritional guidance that can be followed. Gives ideals for how to develop meals based on balance of nutrients and servings from food groups versus specifying eating of "good" versus "bad" foods
- Teaches servings and portion control by focusing on servings and serving sizes, which can teach portion control to those that might overconsume

- Very flexible and allows a wide variety of foods. People who have other dietary restrictions should find it relatively simple to adapt

Cons:

- Diet is very complex. Proportional diets can involve tracking of Calories and Calories per meal, or the grams of macronutrients: carbs, fat, or protein. Tracking that requires multiple calculations to first establish BMR and then the percentage of Calories from each macronutrient before determining grams or determining grams of each macronutrient from one's body weight.
- Sustainability might be an issue because of all the calculations that are required and the consistent weighing and measuring of foods following proportionality diets beyond counting servings per day can be compromised when not cooking one's own meals.

Take-home message:

The use of proportional diets and the concepts of proportionality of nutrients in our diet is a very easy idea to integrate into our daily dietary habits and should be used to develop a balanced dietary strategy. The ideas of balance and proportionality are something that is seen throughout each of the dogmatic diets and might be considered a fundamental principle and foundation to any diet that one might choose to follow.

However, it must be stated clearly and unequivocally that even though we generally talk about diet and food intake based on terms like Caloric density, or the relative difference of Calorie intake from one's BMR, it should not be seen as the foundational value to our diet or our nutrition. Even when we like to cite Calories as being the contributing factor for weight loss or weight maintenance, changes or maintenance of body weight come not from the availability of Calories but from the availability of the nutrients necessary for metabolism. Where lack of nutrients from the diet will be met by removal of tissues of the body that contain that nutrient, and thus nutrient balance may be a larger contributor to weight loss or maintenance. A message that I know is counter to what we have routinely been told but deserves to be the primary focus of future conversations on the topic, as once again the overall idea of Caloric balance may be a misguided ideal.

I need a remedy...

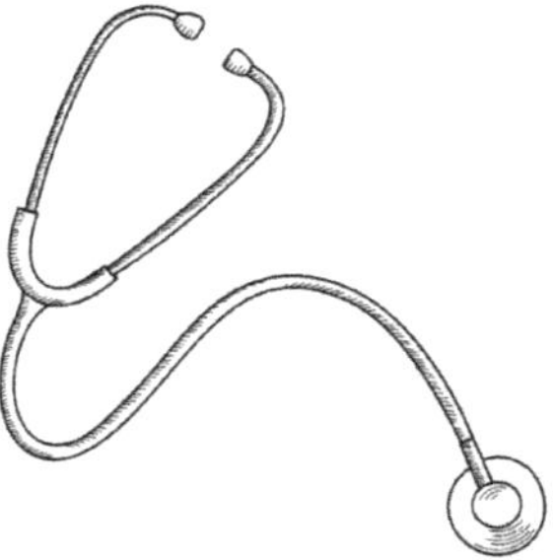

"Let food be thy medicine and medicine be thy food."-
- Attributed to Hippocrates of Kos, c.400 B.C.E.

Beyond the idea of diet to meet religious stipulations, diets have classically been used by physicians as a means to control and possibly cure diseased conditions. Ideals that come from the medical traditions that we trace back to Hippocrates, Galen, and the cult of Asclepius in ancient Greece and Rome that form the foundation for western medical traditions. Concepts that develop the foundation of what we categorize as Oriental medicine and get embedded into discussions regarding superfoods, herbs, and extracts that many faithfully take on a daily basis. Ideals that today have become central to many public health discussions surrounding possible cures to the pandemic of overfatness and obesity that has taken hold over the last half-century.

The premise is that suboptimal nutrition leads to the onset of diseases, leading to remedies that have spawned many of the fad diets that have taken on the guise of religious dogmas being discussed in this book. Yet at the same time, many medical professionals will integrate faddish diets into suggestions, table Diets1, and prescriptions for their patients to follow to alleviate symptoms of diseases, and in some instances as potential cures. Concepts that have spread to nutrition as medicine in the same manner that exercise as medicine has become integrated into holistic medical approaches for chronic and non-communicable diseases.

Table Diets1. Dogmatic diets that have become commonly supported by healthcare professionals to alleviate chronic and non-communicable diseases.

Low Sodium Diet	Low-Calorie Proportional Diet
Low-Fat Diet	Ketogenic (Low Carbohydrate) Diet
Low-Glycemic and High Fiber Diet	Time-Restricted Feeding
Organic Food	Mindful Eating Habits
Vegetarian Diet	Knife-over-fork
Mediterranean Diet	

The largest problem with many of the dietary recommendations that can be offered is the base knowledge of the adviser on diet, nutrition, and its impact on our metabolism. While many of us have become convinced of the importance of food in causing and curing our health problems, many of the healthcare professionals have about the same rudimentary knowledge about nutrition and the impact that nutrition has on metabolism, as we do. Meaning that those we rely upon to give us the best advice about our health are as likely to be susceptible to falling for bias and logical fallacies in making dietary recommendations as anyone else. Where they can be willing to recommend diets that have limited evidence to support the claims of benefit and may be willing to ignore evidence of adverse effects that a given diet might have.

What is interesting is that even with these limitations, we know that with improved nutritional knowledge comes selections of better food choices. A premise within a nutritional dogma for health is that by educating patients about nutrition and nutrition guidelines, they will make better decisions on foods to eat and foods to avoid. Thus, we can view nutrition education as potentially an indoctrination into a specific diet dogma that aligns with the nutrition educator or healthcare professional that is making the recommendations. Something that was seen when dietary practice to health first came to prominence in the late 1800s with the introduction of the plant-based diets marketed by Kellogg and Post in the United States and the nutritional diets developed by Nestle in Europe. Ideas that continue today with the most prominent of the dietary treatments for diseases being the DASH, the low-fat, the low-glycemic diets meant to treat cardiovascular disease and metabolic stresses, while potentially leading to a loss of body weight. Along with the addition of plant, and herbs (or supplements) typically labeled as a group as "superfoods" that should be added to one's typical diet to alleviate metabolic stress independent of any changes in body weight.

DASH Diet and Low-Fat Diet

The DASH (Dietary Approaches to Stop Hypertension) diet is the primary dietary treatment offered by the American Heart Association. The idea and tenets of the DASH diet is centered on the premise that high salt intake is the root cause for high blood pressure and the subsequent heart disease that impacts overall health. Ideas and tenets that arise for medical and public health research from Lewis Dahl beginning in the late 1950s and continuing through the 1970s lead to the public health movements of the 1980s to cut salt from the diet.

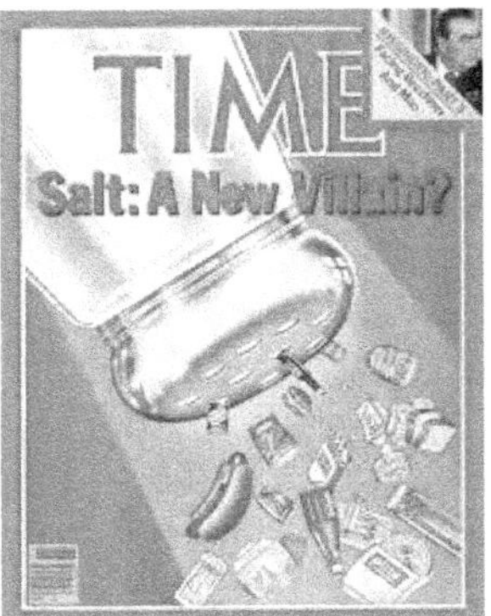

Cover of Time Magazine March 15ᵗʰ, 1982.

If we follow this premise and look at the idealized tenets of the DASH (and the low-fat diet), we are once again following a proportionality diet. Tenets of proportionality that has us shift the proportion of micronutrient (i.e., sodium) and macronutrient (i.e., saturated fat and total fat) intake in the diet that, by reducing sodium and saturated fat, are meant to improve cardiovascular health, while reducing fat intake is meant to lead to weight loss. Based on these generalizations, the DASH diet portrays itself and its dogmas to the followers as a "healthy-eating plan to prevent and treat high blood pressure," by focusing on vegetables, fruits, and whole grains; foods high in minerals l ke potassium, calcium, and magnesium that also include fat-free (or low-fat) cairy products, fish, poultry, beans, and nuts (see table DASH-1). At the same time, the diet restricts fatty meat, full-fat dairy, and processed cereals and grains that are high in sodium, added sugars, and saturated fat. The premise is that by limiting sodium, added sugars, and saturated fats, the diet may help lower low-density lipoprotein (or LDL cholesterol) and extra blood volume that are linked to high blood pressure, increased risk for heart disease, and stroke.

Table DASH-1. Food groups and serving recommendations for following the DASH diet.

Food Group	Servings
Grains	6-to-8 servings a day. 1-serving: ½-cup cooked-cereal, rice or pasta, 1-slice of bread, 1-ounce dry cereal
Vegetables	4-to-5 servings a day. 1-serving: 1-cup raw leafy green vegetable, ½-cup cut-up raw or cooked vegetables, ½-cup (4-Fluid ounces) vegetable juice
Fruits	4-to-5 servings a day. 1-serving: 1-medium fruit, ½-cup fruit (fresh, frozen or canned) fruit, ½-cup (4-Fluid ounces) fruit juice.
Dairy	Fat-Free or Low-fat—Preference toward fat free 2-to-3 servings a day. 1-serving: 1-cup (8-Fluid Ounces) milk or yogurt, 1.5-ounces cheese
Meat	Lean/Low-fat Beef, Poultry, Pork, Lamb, Fish 4-to-6-ounces per day broken up to 1-ounce serving or less per meal 1-serving: 1-ounce of cooked meat, 1-large egg. 1-ounce=28.35 grams
Nuts, Seeds, Beans	4-to-5 servings a week. 1-serving: 1/3-cup nuts, 2-tablespoons peanut butter, 2-tablespoons seeds, ½-cup cooked legumes
Fats and Oils	2-to-3 servings a day 1-serving:1-teaspoon soft margarine, vegetable oil, 1-tablespoon mayonnaise, 2-tablespoons salad dressing
Sweets and Processed Foods	5-servings or fewer a week 1-serving: 1-tablespoon sugar, jelly or jam, ½-cup sorbet, 1-cup sweetened drinks

The DASH diet is really a specific proportionality diet, which means we need to view it similarly to those styles of diets. In this we are given the following general guidelines for following the DASH diet, sodium intake is capped at 2,300 milligrams (2.3 grams) per day versus the 4,000 milligrams (4 grams) that are the normal cap, and fat intake is capped at less than 25% of total caloric intake and saturated fat is capped at less than 5%. Since the focus of the diet is on food low in salt, and to make sure that the low salt tenet is followed it is important to:

- Read food labels and choose low-salt or no-salt-added options.
- Use salt-free spices or flavorings instead of salt.
- Don't add salt when cooking rice, pasta, or hot cereal.
- Choose plain, fresh or frozen vegetables.
- Choose fresh skinless poultry, fish, and lean cuts of meat.

- Eat less restaurant food. When eating at restaurants, ask for dishes with less salt and ask not to have salt added to your order.

A dietary practice that typically gets linked with the DASH diet in treating heart disease is the low-fat diet. The ideals and generalizations of the low-fat diet stem from the public health campaign championed by physician and medical researcher Ancel Keys.

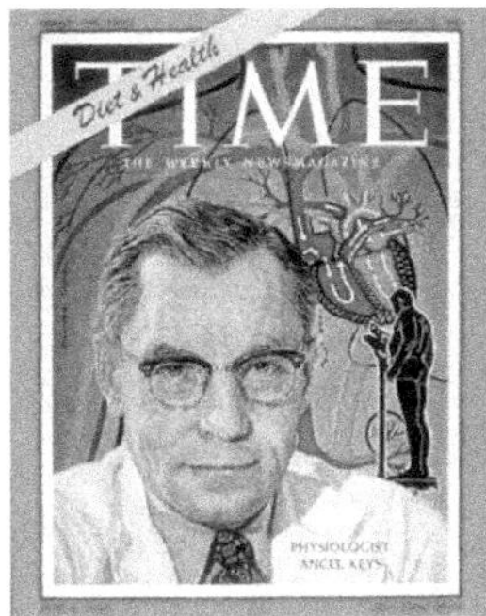

Cover of Time Magazine, January 13ᵗʰ, 1961

The premise on following the low-fat diet is twofold. First, those that consume diets high in fat have a greater risk for heart disease based on several correlational studies relating the composition of foods in one's diet with cardiovascular mortality throughout the population. Correlations that are associated with elevated levels of cholesterol and triglycerides in the blood for those that have a higher fat diet and the negative relationship that these levels have on heart health and blood pressure, but the degree of causality is not entirely present to the point that would allow us to state that the diet is the lone culprit. The second is that fat consumption is associated with gains in body fat and a higher percentage of fat mass. A premise that stems from the misguided notion that weight gain is based on Calories that one eats and that fat has the greatest Calorie value of the macronutrients that we view from an energy standpoint. A viewpoint on Calories that is correct, even if flawed as it relates to body composition and weight, will be the rationale that acolytes of the low-fat dietary approach will voice, even if there is limited evidence to support the viewpoint and that weight gain or loss is highly complex based on a host of interacting factors that lead to growth or loss of tissue that is not dependent on Calories.

From these premises the dogma of low-fat has taken hold, taken hold not only within those that practice this dogmatic dietary practice but also throughout conversation about fat and fat content in specific foods or meals that we have throughout society.

Just think about how one might talk about the "grease" that is seen on a pizza, or how worse it is to eat a fast-food hamburger versus a meatball sandwich. Even if the nutritional content of the sandwich and the hamburger are exactly the same and there are actually fewer Calories in the hamburger relative to the sandwich for those that adhere to this misnomer on Calories and body weight. A similar conversation takes hold when discussing the cooking methods and the need to use your air fryer and not oil fry your foods, based on the addition of adding fat to the fried foods. While there is some indication that frying in oil can add metabolic disruptors (pyrolyzed hydrocarbons) to food, the general conversation that takes place is about the additional fat and "Calories" that comes from the frying in oil and not the potential metabolic effect that pyrolyzed-hydrocarbons might have on our body.

At the same time, the conversations stemming from the low-fat diets have led to conversations about foods with "good" fats versus foods with "bad" fats, conversations that parallel the conversations about sugars and carbohydrates that have become more commonplace with growing awareness of low-carbohydrate and low-glycemic diets. Where "good" fats typically are the polyunsaturated and monounsaturated fats obtained from vegetable oils or the monounsaturated fats that are identified as the omega-3 or omega-6 fats. These "good" monounsaturated fats will sometimes get labeled as the "healthy" fats or the "heart-healthy" fats on a lot of the packed foods we buy. While "bad" fats are the saturated fats, they are not any saturated fats...

only the saturated fats coming from animal-based products or meats and not the saturated fats coming from nuts or seeds.

We further define the low-fat diet to be a diet where fat contributes no more than 11-20% of total Calories in a day, with saturated fat contributing 2-5% of total Calories, versus the reduced fat consumption that is followed by the DASH diet, where fat consumption is capped at a Caloric contribution of 25% total and 5% from saturated fats. This general rule has been expanded to the packaged foods we see being labeled as low-fat or "lite" when the packed food provides 100 calories and it has 3 grams or less of fat within a serving. Based on the tenets of the low-fat dogma, the following guidelines can be offered regarding food choices and cooking methods:

Fat
- Limit total intake of fats and oils, along with limiting saturated fats and trans fats in the diet by avoiding butter, stick margarine, shortening, lard, palm, and coconut oil
- Choose low-fat, non-hydrogenated fats and nonfat options for mayonnaise, peanut butter, salad dressings, gravy, or condiments
- Choose vegetable oil, e.g., canola or sunflower oil, or olive oil
- Use nuts in moderation
- Avoid high-fat processed, and convenience foods

Meats and Meat Alternatives
- Choose fish, chicken, turkey, and lean meats insteac of fatty meats, pork or beef. If you eat red meat, or pork, limit to 3 servings per week and choose "leanest cuts"
- Use dried beans, peas, lentils, and tofu instead of animal proteins
- Choose egg whites over whole eggs and limit egg yolks to 4-yolks per week at most
- Avoid fatty meats, such as bacon, sausage, franks, luncheon meats, and ribs, and all organ meats, including liver.

Dairy
- Choose lower fat (1% or skim) or non-fat milk, yogurt and cottage cheese, and cheeses made
- Avoid high-fat and hard cheeses
- Choose 1%, skim, or fat-free cream

Fruits and Vegetables

- Eat a variety of fruits and vegetables with high fiber content
- Use alternatives to fats to increase the palatability of vegetables (e.g., lemon juice, vinegar, or "mist" olive oil dressing)

Breads, Cereals and Grains

- Choose whole-grain breads, cereals, pastas, and rice.
- Avoid high-fat and processed snacks, breads, or desserts (e.g., cakes, cookies, croissants, doughnuts, granola, muffins, pastries, pies).

Cooking Tips

- Trim visible fat off meats and remove skin from poultry before cooking.
- Bake, broil, boil, poach, or roast when cooking poultry, fish, and lean meats
- Avoid fried foods and drain fat from meat as you cook it.
- Add little or no fat to foods and use vegetable oil sprays to grease pans for cooking or baking.
- Steam vegetables.
- Use herbs and no-oil marinades to increase the palatability of foods

What benefits do we get from the DASH and low-fat diets?

Based on the evidence we have; the DASH diet has the potential to lower blood pressure and reduce blood lipid levels that lead to an improvement in heart health. Along with reducing blood pressure and improving heart health, the DASH diet has been linked with reduced body weight and fat mass, alleviates metabolic syndrome and type-2 diabetes, and reduces the relative risk for cancer. Benefits attributed to the diet are linked with increased consumption of fiber, potassium, magnesium, and calcium, along with increased levels of polyphenols, carotenoids, and phytosterols coming from higher intake of fruits, vegetables, and whole grains found in the diet. Leading to greater levels of flavonoids, β-carotene, β-cryptoxanthin, lycopene, lutein+zeaxanthin that reduce the impact on oxidative stress and lower the level of inflammation and help alleviate symptoms of metabolic diseases associated with overfatness and obesity.

However, these benefits appear to be attributed to high adherence to the diet and its dogmatic tenets of low sodium, low fat, and low sugar. Additionally, the potential to have responses appears to be linked to the "sensitivity" that someone has to salt intake along with co-morbidity (e.g., age, gender, smoking history, level of physical activity). Where those who are older, highly sedentary, and have the greatest reduction in salt and fluid intake have the greatest response, while those that are young and active tend to have limited responses. What is also interesting is that non-white adults (regardless of age) tend to see greater improvements in blood pressure and heart health, yet there is not a scientifically valid rationale as the only hypothesis offered is an outdated and nullified hypothesis that sensitivity to salt varies in people based on socially recognized ethnicity. Based on the degree of reduction in sugars and total nutrient balance (as determined by Caloric restriction), there is a noted change in lifespan for rodents, something that we don't have evidence to state is true for people.

Along with many of the benefits associated with the DASH diet, low-fat diets have also been associated with weight loss and loss of fat mass, especially in the very short-term. Weight loss that is accompanied by improvements in heart health and reduced blood pressures that are linked to reduced levels of LDL and cholesterol can occur independent of changes in body weight and could be linked with reduced consumption of animal-derived proteins and the antigens that can trigger atherosclerosis. Along with improved heart health, low-fat diets are associated with reduced risk for certain cancers and metabolic syndrome (type-2 diabetes), which appears to be associated with reduced consumption of cooked animal proteins and pyrolyzed hydrocarbons that can act like metabolic disruptors.

What are the costs and risks that might come from following the tenets of the DASH and low-fat diets?
The DASH diet tends to be well tolerated by most individuals. However, the premise of following the DASH diet can compromise exercise performance

and may lead to issues associated with dehydration (i.e., cramping, fatigue). The restriction of sodium, a major factor in drawing water into the body, can impact the ability to reach and then maintain a normal hydration. Meaning that those who are following secondary recommendations for increased exercise to treat high blood pressure may need more salt in their diet than permitted by the DASH guidelines to prevent a reduction in performance of cramping. The hydration issue can also be an issue for anyone that utilizes diuretics in combination with the DASH diet independent of additional exercise, as the medication makes it even more difficult to retain fluids to ensure hydration is normal.

Outside of the issue with sodium and hydration, the consumption of large amounts of plant-based foods increases the anti-nutrients that can also impact the bioavailability of many ions, impacting normal metabolic activity at various tissues of the body. While there are indications for reduced risks for kidney stones, the interactions of anti-nutrients on Calcium movement may actually increase the risk. An increased risk that can become more problematic given how the diet may impact normal hydration and how that impact can negatively influence kidney functions.

Beyond these factors, the general premise and ideals that form the foundational tenets for following the DASH diet have logical flaws that need to be addressed. The idea that salt and the amount of salt in the diet is the root cause of hypertension is a generalization that does not hold true. The methods of research used were flawed as if these were observation studies and not controlled studies that used correlative association to draw conclusions. Meaning that there are a host of factors that contribute to blood pressure and heart health that were ignored and measures that were seen as outliers were ignored, even though the responses fell within the range for what we deem a normal responses. These flaws in methods call into question the validity of the conclusions and whether or not high salt diets actually contribute to the blood pressure issues that the proponents of the diet claim the diet will cure. There is also an issue with the populations that were used in the initial research that was used to formulate the diet and subsequent cohort studies to validate the use of the diet. The populations were extremely selective and very small, and given the multitudes of factors that come into play as it relates to cardiovascular health, the choice of people to include in the studies, just like the methods, calls into question the general premise that served to form the hypothesis about salt and high blood pressure along with the primary tenet that guides the DASH diet. The last comment that needs to be made related to the questionable research methods is that following the observational studies, the guise for developing the DASH diet and the reduced sodium intake is entirely justified through rodent studies and not human-controlled studies.

The premise of following a low-fat diet stems from studies touted by Ancel Keys that stipulated diets high in fat and cholesterol lead to heart disease while suggesting that low-fat diets prevent heart disease. Leading to public health promotion of the low-fat diets by the 1980s for everyone as a way to not only prevent heart disease but also as a means to mitigate a growing population of overweight individuals, an ideology that became a central dietary tenet for healthcare professionals and advocacy agencies, health and fitness influencers, and the population altogether. Yet, there is no evidence to support either Keys' zealousness for the low-fat diet or the ideological fervor that many healthcare professionals pitch such a diet to their patients. Additionally, greater understanding of metabolic functions has led to acknowledgment that overfatness and obesity are not dependent on fat content in one's diet. Moreover, the bliss point response and palatability of food mean we need to add sweeteners and sugars to the foods that have had fat removed. Additions of chemicals that are independent of hormone regulation lead to the accumulation of fat in adipose tissue, greater body fat, and the adverse health effects of overfatness that were meant to be alleviated by the low-fat diet. Nevertheless, countering this effect feels like Sisyphus pushing the boulder up the mountain, as even with evidence to show the downsides of the low-fat diet are greater than the benefits, the ideology has become more entrenched, and the skepticism is generally dismissed.

Both DASH and low-fat diets, like many of the various dogmatic diets, can lead to nutrient deficiencies. Low-fat diets can lead to deficiencies in total fat, especially in essential fatty-acids (ALA, EPA, DHA) along with fat-soluble vitamins (vitamin A, D, E, K). The deficiencies in fat and fat-soluble nutrients have adverse impacts on health and performance, including poor neurological function and potential psychosis, compromised metabolic health and reduced insulin sensitivity, increased oxidative stress and inflammation, compromised hormone production (i.e., steroid hormones), and altered reward responses with possible anxiety or depression.

Due to the restrictiveness of the diets, the rate of compliance and adherence for both the DASH and the low-fat diets tends to be low. While the commercialization of the low-fat diet has become mainstream, allowing for pre-packaged and restaurant options, the same cannot be said for the DASH diet, making it incredibly hard for those following a DASH diet to eat outside the home without complicating ordering or finding foods with lower sodium content (which recently has become more prevalent for certain salted snacks). There may also be low compliance and adherence for the DASH diet due to the palatability of food, since salt is a major flavor enhancer, while low-fat diet foods can have excess sugar and sweetness to the foods that are meant to make the foods more palatable but may take foods beyond the bliss point for enjoyment. The impact on compliance and adherence becomes more pronounced when it is followed for longer durations without consistent coercion or reinforcement.

And it has only been recently that we started to question the validity of adhering to the low-fat diets, as evidence has begun to surface regarding the impact that fats and sugars have on metabolism, oxidative stress, and overall health. Evidence that has been provided by the other excessively popular medical diet dogma, the low-glycemic and low-carbohydrate diets used in the treatment of diabetes.

Low-Glycemic Diet (Diabetic Diet)

Given the current pandemic of overfatness and metabolic disease that faces humanity, the diet dogma that is discussed and followed, sometimes without awareness, is the low-glycemic or diabetic diet. Think about how often you hear people talk about food that "spikes Insulin" or foods that have "hidden sugars" in them. Just like how the low-fat craze changed how we discuss fat in our diets, the low-glycemic diets have changed how we discuss carbohydrates and sugars in our diet. The premise of the diet is based on observations that societies that had a dietary focus on consuming whole grains, legumes, and nuts (low glycemic index foods) had a lower prevalence of metabolic diseases or overfatness, while those societies that shifted their diet to highly processed and sugary foods had a dramatically higher prevalence of metabolic disease or overfatness. Where the central tenet is that if we are able to control glycemic responses from foods, then we can avert overfatness or metabolic diseases.

The low-glycemic or diabetic diet is a dietary practice that focuses on foods that would lower total carbohydrate load through focusing on foods with more fiber and less total carbohydrates. The idea of the diet is based on the premise of the glycemic index, a method that ranks foods from 1 to 100 according to how much they affect a person's blood sugar, where pure glucose provides a reference score of 100 and ranking of foods is identified as **high** (where foods score above 70), **medium** (where the food scores between 56 and 69), and **low** (where foods score less than 55). With the premise that by consuming foods based on awareness of the glycemic index, people are able to choose foods that are lower in sugar and carbohydrates, table LCD-1. Selections that can in turn help people who want to lose weight or manage conditions such as diabetes.

Table LCD-1. Commonly consumed foods and the average glycemic index for each food.—source American Diabetic Association.

High Glycemic Index Foods (>70)	Medium Glycemic Index Foods (56-69)	Low Glycemic Index Foods (<55)
Glucose (103)	Wheat flake biscuits (69)	Specialty grain bread (53)
Potato, instant mash (87)	Brown rice, boiled (68)	Rice noodles (53)
Rice crackers/crisps (87)	Millet porridge (67)	Taro, boiled (53)
Rice milk (86)	Couscous (65)	Chapati (52)
Cornflakes (81)	Popcorn (65)	Sweet corn (52)
Instant oat porridge (79)	Sucrose (65)	Banana, raw (51)
Rice porridge/congee (78)	Pumpkin, boiled (64)	Ice cream (51)
Potato, boiled (78)	Potato, French fries (63)	Mango, raw (51)
Watermelon, raw (76)	Sweet potato, boiled (63)	Orange juice (50)
White wheat bread (75)	Wheat roti (62)	Spaghetti, white (49)
Whole wheat bread (74)	Honey (61)	Strawberry jam (49)
White rice, boiled (73)	Soft drink/soda (59)	Vegetable soup (48)
Unleavened wheat bread (70)	Pineapple, raw (59)	Spaghetti, whole meal (48)
	Muesli (57)	Corn tortilla (46)
	Potato crisps (56)	Dates, raw (42)
	Plantain/green banana (55)	Peaches, canned (43)
	Udon noodles (55)	Orange, raw (43)
	Porridge, rolled oats (55)	Yogurt, fruit (41)
		Apple juice (41)
		Chocolate (40)
		Milk, full fat (39)
		Carrots, boiled (39)
		Milk, skim (37)
		Apple, raw (36)
		Soy milk (34)
		Lentils (32)
		Barley (28)
		Chickpeas (28)
		Kidney beans (24)
		Soya beans (16)
		Fructose (15)

Another measurement is the glycemic load that comes from the foods that we are eating. This value is a reflection not of the impact that the food has on glucose levels in the blood but of the portion of food coming from carbohydrates. However, it is important that many healthcare professionals have begun to question the advice of the glycemic index and glycemic load because of the complexity in determining scores and load along with variability in values that any single food might have based on where a person looks. This is where we get a secondary diet dogma stemming from the diabetic diet, the low-carbohydrate diet that looks at total grams of carbohydrates and not necessarily the glycemic load. With an appreciation of many that this value is actually more important at revising issues of overfatness and metabolic diseases than the glycemic index values. A premise that has led many proponents of the low-glycemic diets to become proponents of the low-carbohydrate diets instead (see "We don't need no stinking carbohydrates" for more on this dogma).

When viewing the glycemic index and following the premise and tenets of the low-glycemic or diabetic diet, is it important to understand what impact the index value has on foods being eaten? The scores that foods get are impacted by the proportionality and ratio of macronutrients (carbohydrates-to-lipids (fats)-to-proteins) in the food and within carbohydrates the amount of fiber relative to total carbohydrates, along with the degree of processing that has taken place in preparing the foods with processed foods having higher values than raw or whole food, and lastly the presence of anti-nutrients and cooking that can impact the availability of nutrients in the foods.

What benefits might come from following the low-glycemic (diabetic) diet?

There is a consensus that the low-glycemic (diabetic) diet has a potential benefit for alleviating symptoms of type 2-diabetes and metabolic syndrome, reduced the risk of developing heart disease, and preventing the issues of overfatness. There is speculation in the consensus that the diet may also provide for a reduced risk for cancer and may potentially provide a means to lose weight.

The primary method of action that has been offered for the diet performing these benefits is through improvement in metabolic health through normalization of Insulin, Glucagon and GLP-1 independent of any changes in glycemia or total carbohydrates being consumed. Additionally, there are changes noted in fat cell metabolism that reduce hormones from the adipose tissue that lead to a reduction in inflammation that furthers the normalizing of metabolic health. When combined with reduced total carbohydrate intake, there can be weight loss that will predominantly come from fat mass due to both metabolic and hormonal changes that are taking place through reduction of sugar intake. Even without reductions in total carbohydrate intake, a reduced glycemic load is associated with reduced oxidative stress and ROS damage.

Improvements in metabolic health can have a positive impact on cardiovascular functions; the higher level of fiber and plant-based foods helps to reduce inflammation that leads to lower blood pressures that allow for the improvement in heart health. Changes are typically linked with reduced levels of C-reactive protein, lower inflammatory adipokines (fat cell hormones), and a reduction in stress hormones that lowers atherosclerosis changes in the blood vessels. These changes also lower heart rate and with lower pressures allow for a more effective heart contraction.

Neurologically, there is an increase in Insulin sensitivity and a reduction in ROS damage that allows for improved function of the neurons in the brain. Improvements that allow for neuron growth and stronger connections between neurons. Changes that lead to improved cognitive functions, improvements in mood and reduction in anxiety, and the reduction in glycemic load can also impact reward center actions and lead to a reduction in addictive eating behaviors and binge eating.

The low-glycemic (diabetic) diet is a proportional diet and thus does not conflict with dietary advice that most of us have heard about throughout our lives and utilizes a combination of servings and food amounts in the recommendations being offered. This makes the diet easy to follow relative to other carbohydrate-restricting diets, especially when applied in the context of healthy diet, healthy food and nutrient-based advice. Additionally, the diet provides knowledge about the quality and amount of carbohydrates we find in the foods we eat and the importance of knowing these values if we wish to reduce non-communicable diseases and promote healthy body composition.

What costs and risks might develop from following a low-glycemic diet?

There are two major limitations that might impact the ability for the low-glycemic (diabetic) diet to be beneficial. First, because the diet is based on keeping index scores low for all foods being eaten and does not specifically eliminate foods from one's diet, we have potential sites for confusion between what we believe are healthier food choices, i.e., French fries have a lower index score relative to baked potatoes even though we view one as unhealthy (French fries) and one as healthy (baked potatoes). Likewise, since there is also no limitation to types of food in the diet and it can very easily include foods (i.e., some processed chocolate treats and low-fat ice cream) that have index scores that are "low" but potentially contain metabolic disruptors that can inhibit any potential benefit arising from following the low-glycemic (diabetic) diet.

Figure 1. The impact that metabolic disruptors have on food intake and metabolic health.

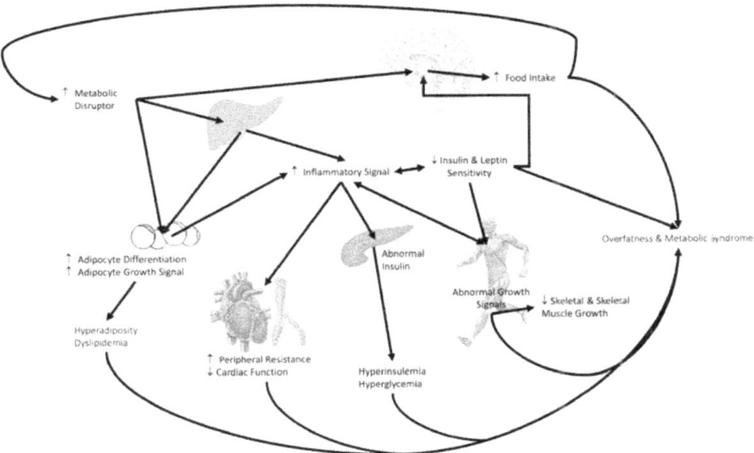

Along with these drawbacks, the second major limitation is seen with increased consumption of plant-based foods suggested by the proponents of the diet. With greater plant-based foods come relatively higher amounts of anti-nutrients being consumed. Increased amounts of anti-nutrients (i.e., phytates, oxalates, tannins, lectins, protease inhibitors) impact the absorption of nutrients from foods being digested and secondarily can impact the bioavailability of nutrients at the cells and tissues of body.

Beyond these major drawbacks, the low-glycemic (diabetic) diet does not consider the total carbohydrate load in the diet. And it is important that when viewing the low-glycemic diet, the index provides an inclination for how quickly glucose might be seen in the bloodstream but does not provide any insight into what might happen metabolically once the carbohydrates get digested and absorbed. Combined with the complexity of following the index for foods it can lead to a diet that is not only difficult to follow and understand or provide the changes in nutrients to change metabolism, allowing for improvement in overall metabolic health or body weight (should body weight be a measure used as a reinforcement for continuing the diet).

What can we say about the diet dogmas (DASH, Low-fat, Low-glycemic or Diabetic diet) developed for health purposes?

For given populations, the use of the DASH, low-fat, or low-glycemic diets can be beneficial. Since the diets were developed for use in a clinical setting, we have ample clinical, observational, and basic science (i.e., cellular and animal model) research to support many of the opinions that are voiced both in favor of and against use of any of these diets. Additionally, the diets are based on primary guides of the proportionality diets, which means it can be easy to follow if guides are provided as general recommendations. Outside of limiting animal-derived foods and total sodium, and in some cases specific carbohydrate-rich foods, the diets tend to be focused on servings and serving sizes versus eating specific types of foods that we see in many of the other dogmas.

Pros

- Reduces metabolic syndrome and improves Insulin and Leptin sensitivity, allowing for a more normal metabolic status and inflammation response
- Improved cardiometabolic health that includes reduced blood pressure and improved heart health along with reduced inflammation and better immune function that negates any symptoms of overfatness from being expressed
- Weight loss, at least in the short term. There is a reduction n both total weight and fat mass in the short term when following any of the diets
- Reduced relative risk for cancer that stems from the imoroved cardiometabolic health and reduction in consumption of metabolic disruptors by limiting the amount of processed foods found in the diet and replacing them with additional low-glycemic and high-fiber fruits and vegetables

Cons

- Complex diets. All of the diets mean needing to track foods and count values found within foods that are being eaten. Because of the complexity, each meal takes planning to remain within limits being set for restriction on macronutrients (e.g., carbohydrate and glycemic load, fat) or micronutrients (e.g., sodium, potassium)
- Costs of following the diet. There is a higher cost to groceries (with poor availability and quality of fruits, vegetables, and lean meats) along with extra fees being added for special menu options when eating at restaurants to replace foods not allowed on the diet with appropriate foods.
- Lack of familiarity with menus and recipes leads to generic foods that are not universally palatable or appealing.
- Restrictive and socially exclusionary limited food options and differences with culturally accepted options can make diet hard to follow for long periods of time.
- Low-fat diets can lead to deficiencies in essential fatty-acids and fat-soluble vitamins necessary for heart and brain health. Additionally, the excess sugar to make foods palatable can lead to weight gain and possibly impact metabolic health.

Take home message on the DASH, Low-Fat, and Low-Glycemic diets:

The medically developed diets can be thought of as proportional diets that do not specify eating special or specific foods, instead providing nutritional goals to limit intake of nutrients that might have previously been ingested in excess. These plans focus on modifying the food groups to increase eating low-glycemic and high-fiber vegetables, fruits, and whole grains, and the elimination of sugar-sweetened beverages and sweets. The DASH and low-fat diets also include a focus on skim (non-fat) or 1% (low-fat) dairy products and lean meats (fish, poultry) with the use of meat alternatives (beans, nuts, and legumes) while limiting oils and fats used in cooking. While the low-glycemic (Diabetic diets) may not place any limits on the fats in diet. While the diets can be tolerated, the restrictiveness of the diets and the social exclusion that might come from following such a diet may make it difficult to follow over the long-term without consistent external feedback and motivation or self-monitoring and self-motivation desire to continue.

"Superfoods"

Before delving into the general premise upholding the dogma of the superfoods, it is important that we answer one burning question: *what are superfoods*? Well, here's the thing; indicating foods as being **superfoods** is really just a marketing gimmick. A message meant to convey that there is some powerful food with a special ability to promote weight loss or heal a worrisome disease. It's a statement meant to increase the marketability of selected and ever-changing lists of foods based on the supposed benefits that you might get from eating specific types of foods, table S1. Marketing that started with the promotion of bananas and carrots to the most recent marketing of nutritional yeasts, bone broths, and collagen powders.

While sold as being scientifically based with the premise by those that follow the superfood dogma that there is science behind their arguments, it needs to be stated that we do not have a scientifically based or regulated definition for what it means to be a superfood. But generally, a food is promoted to superfood status when it offers high levels of desirable nutrients, is linked to the prevention of a disease, or is believed to offer several simultaneous health benefits beyond its nutritional value. However, one value that we see across foods bragged about as being supe-food is distinct antioxidant properties that might give benefits to a person in need of additional antioxidants, table S2.

Table S1. List of some of the historically viewed superfoods, in alphabetical order. List is non-exhaustive as indication of superfood is constantly changing

Foods A-J	Foods K-Z
Acai	Kale
Almonds	Kimchi
Artichoke	Legumes (Chickpea, Lentils, Peas and
Avocado	Pea protein, Soybeans)
Arugula	Leafy Greens (Chards, Dandelions,
Banana	Beets, Lettuce, Turnip)
Barley	Maca
Berries (Raspberry, Strawberry,	Mango
Blueberry, Cranberry, Blackberry)	Onion
Buckwheat	Oregano
Cacao and Dark Chocolate	Peppermint
Carrots	Pineapple
Cassava	Pomegranate
Cashew	Quinoa
Cherry	Rosemary
Chia	Salmon, Trout, Tuna
Cinnamon	Seaweed
Coconut (and Oil)	Sorghum
Coffee (Green Coffee)	Spelt
Cruciferous vegetable (Broccoli,	Spinach
Cauliflower)	Stone Fruits
Eggs	Sunflower seed
Fermented Dairy (Yogurt, Kefir)	Sweet Potato
Fish (Mackerel, Herring, Sardines,	Tea (Green Tea)
Anchovies)	Teff
Flax seed (and Oil)	Thyme
Garlic	Turmeric
Ginger	Walnuts
Goji	Wheatgrass
Grape seed	
Hemp seed (and Oil)	

When we discuss these superfoods, it means needing to understand chemical reactions known as reduction and oxidation reactions, simplified to RedOx reactions, that take place in every cell of our body. These reactions occur during metabolic reactions when electrons are moving between atoms in the molecules being formed or broken. In these reactions, reduction indicates gaining an electron in the molecule, making it a "reduced" molecule, while oxidation indicates losing an electron in the molecule, making it an "oxidized" molecule. When a molecule gets oxidized we tend to add a new term, calling it a "free radical" or a "reactive oxidative species," sometimes simply called ROS. These oxidized molecules then go about reacting with every molecule that they come in contact with, trying to become stable (regain the missing electron), and with every interaction that the molecule has, it causes small molecular damage to the cells that can quickly add up and lead to oxidative injury. The oxidative injury is what gets labeled as oxidative stress. To counter these free radicals, our cells will generate a molecule that can interact without getting damaged, antioxidants.

Table S2. Commonly recognized antioxidants found within the food sources that might be considered as "superfood" in the context of dogmatic diets.

Vitamin and Coenzyme Antioxidant	Other Antioxidants
	Branched-chain Amino Acids
Vitamin A	Omega-3 Fatty Acids
Vitamin B_2 (Riboflavin)	Carotenoids
Vitamin B_3 (Niacin)	Flavonoid
Vitamin B_6 (Pyridoxine)	Glutathione
Vitamin B_9 (Folate)	Phenolic Compounds
Vitamin B_{12} (Cobalamin)	Phytochemicals and Phytosterols
Vitamin D	Copper
Vitamin C	Magnesium
Vitamin E	Manganese
Co-Q_{10}	Selenium
	Zinc

We all need antioxidants in our diet to help with the antioxidants that the body is normally producing on a daily basis. And this is where the proponents of this dogmatic diet will find their rationale. When there is an increase in oxidative stress, a situation where free radicals are being formed more quickly than the antioxidants are able to neutralize them, then we need even more antioxidants in our diet. These situations occur when we are stressed, have inflammatory responses, get exposed to environmental toxins, or exposed to cigarette smoke, drink alcohol, or have metabolites formed from a diet that is high in simple sugars (e.g., sucrose, fructose). If we look at this list, proponents of this dietary dogma state, "hey, this is modern life, and we need superfoods to help with modern life." Where the followers of the superfood dogma rationalize following the dogma as a way to delay the aging effects of modern life. Because regardless of the root cause, if I have too much oxidative stress then I start to express and experience "aging." All of the classic signs that we typically think about when we think about "aging" for someone (e.g., lapses of memory, graying of hair, wrinkles) come from oxidative stress.

Which leads to the question, what evidence do we have to support the use of superfoods?

To address this question, it is important to understand claims are frequently not strongly supported by scientific evidence, which has led to that ever-growing list of superfoods that typically goes unchecked. The lack of established criteria and limited evidence has provided rationale that claims of superfood should be considered more as "food fraud." However, there are some recognized benefits from different types of superfoods based on the level of oxidative stress that one might have. Most of these benefits come from extrapolation of animal studies on longevity and chemical analysis of the foods to determine the quantity and quality of the antioxidant compounds that are contained within the samples.

There are a lot of correlative studies that support the consumption of many superfoods. The primary associated factors to support the consumption come from acquiring vitamins and coenzymes involved with limiting the formation of free radicals or the elimination of radicals once they are formed. Most of the fruits and vegetables also provide many minerals used in elimination reactions of the radicals, while the proteins found in many of the fermented foods, eggs, fruits, and vegetables provide amino acids necessary for the elimination of toxins by the liver and kidney. At the same time the phytosterols and phytochemicals from the plants are associated with altering hormonal signals that can reduce blood pressure and improvement in glucose metabolism. The fermented beverages can also act as seeding agents of microbiome within the intestines that can help with generating a "healthier" microbiome in our intestines. Changes in the microbiome toward "healthier" for those that have a compromised microbiome have been associated with improvements in inflammation and immune responses along with reduced overall oxidative stress.

If we were to view all of the limited studies in total, there appears to be a correlative reduced relative risk for developing cancers, cardiovascular disease, dementia, and metabolic syndrome for those that consume superfoods with limits to the total volume of foods consumed.

So, we don't have a lot of evidence for benefit; is there anything to worry about?

One of the largest problems related to the superfood dogmatic diet is in how they are consumed. These "superfoods" are sold as some sort of tablet or powder, with the idea that by drinking juice containing the extracts from a "superfood," you will gain nutritional support that would be obtained from eating that same food. Yet, eating food means getting greater total nutritional value versus what can be obtained from grinding up that food or taking it as an elixir in a capsule; the benefit that I could get from that specific food drops. Then there are some superfoods where processing of the food source is necessary to extract the beneficial chemicals. Things that we turn into beverages, soups, or teas have their antioxidant properties expressed that would not be present without the processing. Yet, for most of the other things that we label as being superfoods, this is not the case; most of the nutritional value that we see from superfoods comes from them being in their "whole food" source, not in their products.

Additionally, we need to remember the idea of bioavailability and bioreactivity that chemicals might have in our body. Bioavailability, is the ability for the nutrient to be processed during digestion and absorption that allows the cells to be able to take it in. Bioreactivity, is the indication that the available molecules have areas of the molecules that are functional and can be used by the cells in their metabolic process. Based on these two factors, it is important that simply seeing individual chemical compounds in foods that have the potential for producing a physiological response does not mean that it will automatically produce that response. As the chemicals present in food or food products will be processed by the cells of the intestine and the liver, that can change how active the molecule will be for the body. Additionally, the amount we are receiving from our foods might not rise to a level that would cause a response; we are not getting a recommended dose.

Something that can be extended to the proponents of superfoods like cinnamon being able to cure diabetes: while cinnamon has an antioxidant and anti-inflammatory compound, the amount consumed in a serving of cinnamon is excessively small, and the activity of the molecule in regulating glucose metabolism is non-existent outside of possibly controlling the inflammation that inhibits normal insulin regulation.

We also must remember something very important about all of this... the baby bear effect. We don't want too much, we don't want too little, we want just right. When taking excessive amounts of antioxidants based on the premise that we are controlling oxidative stress, we can actually cause oxidative stress to occur. This happens when the antioxidant molecule starts acting like a free radical and causes oxidative stress through the formation of oxidized molecules.

The other is also a caution that we need to have related to the superfood labeling and the superfood dogmatic diets; there is very limited empirical evidence to support many of the claims that are out there. And when we do see peer-reviewed research on these superfoods, most study designs have at least one flaw in their methodology or in their analysis of results that can very easily call into question the conclusions being inferred. Flaws that limit how much we can take away from the conclusions and claims of benefits about consuming these superfoods.

Take-home message on superfoods

We want to imagine foods can have special abilities for our health. Foods and supplements that have the ability to promote weight loss. Have the ability to heal our bodies and cure diseases. It is important that while we talk about "superfoods" and the term is present in the dictionary, that is not the same as having evidence of its effectiveness. There is no scientifically based rationale for claiming foods to be "super," and scientifically there is no consensus for the definition of superfood. Yet, a food gets promoted to superfood status when it offers high levels of desirable nutrients, gets linked with disease prevention, or offers health benefits beyond what can be found from the nutritional value of the food. Most foods that we see as being claimed to be superfoods are those that contain antioxidants that have some potential benefit, but in high concentrations can have an adverse impact on our overall health.

The use of the term in marketing of foods and supplements can cause blindness to food options. Focusing on a few selected foods that are thought to be "superfoods" can lead people to omit or ignore foods that offer equal benefits with greater nutrient loads that are missing in the supposed superfood. The blinding to foods can limit the variety of foods in the diet that is important not only to provide the wide array of micronutrients necessary for normal metabolism but will also help prevent overconsumption of any specific nutrient or limit the likelihood of becoming bored with one's diet.

Carbs... we don't need no stinking Carbs...

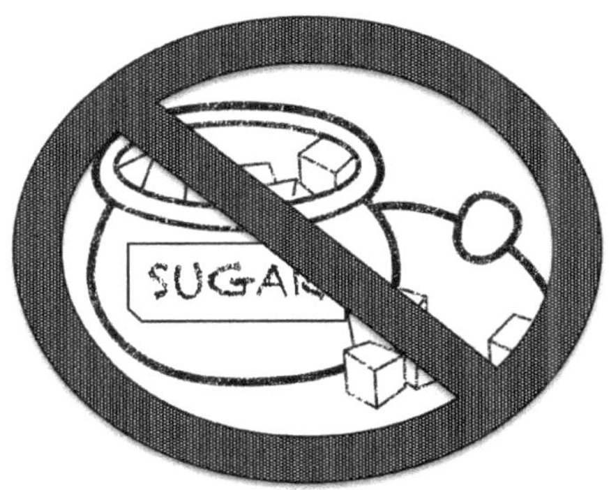

If we were to look historically at the faddish diets that originated from the medical community meant to treat a host of metabolic diseases and possibly encourage weight loss, we need to look no further than the low-carbohydrate diets. The various versions of low-carbohydrate diets have taken a number of different views over the nearly two centuries since first published in the mid-1800s by Bernard Moncriff in *An Exclusively Animal Diet* (1856), William Banting as the diet he followed for weight loss in his *Letter on Corpulence* published in Harper's Weekly (1862), and subsequent diets put forth by physicians Cantini and Salisbury in the 1870s and 1880s. It was with Cantini's and Salisbury's suggestions that a diet of all meat and hot water can alleviate many maladies of our health that we see the birth of the low-carb/high-protein diets of today. It is the low-carbohydrate dietary advice that has been used throughout medical history, by hosts of physicians, for treating diabetic patients as a means to control blood glucose levels and diabetic conditions.

These premises and medical advice have become exceedingly popular in the context of general dietary conversations and advertisements as we seek ways to control glucose and Insulin spikes that might come from sugars in our diets. Dietary advice has also taken hold through the adage of minimizing "added" sugars in our diet based on the premise that sugar in the diet is somehow the bane of our overall health. Conversations about nutrients in the diet over the last couple of decades not only stipulated that we should avoid sugars at all costs but at the same time discussed carbohydrates as being either "good" or "bad" sugars, while simultaneously offering the adage that we need more protein in our diet. Discussions that lead to the dogmatic practice of the very-low carbohydrate trinity of "keto diet," "paleo diet," and the "carnivore diet."

Atkins and Ketogenic Diets

We might have already heard of the ketogenic diet, or "going keto" as it is commonly referred to, as it has become a very popular branch of the dogmatic diet. But what is the ketogenic diet? A lot will preach this as being the "Atkins" diet, as Dr. Atkins famously prophesied the health benefits of eating this way. While others simply refer to it as a "low carb" diet. The ketogenic diet is similar to the diabetic diet or the low-glycemic index diets but is also very different. The diabetic diet reduces starchy foods and foods with added sugars but does not specifically advise for increases in proteins or fats to offset the reduction in the starchy carbohydrates.

Whatever you wish to call it, the ketogenic diet is a diet that is meant to eliminate a lot of the sugars and starches and replace them primarily with fats in the diet, but some styles of keto diets have one increase their protein intake along with a slight increase in fats. So, depending upon what type of ketogenic diet you might follow, you'll see a different type of breakdown in terms of fats versus protein.

Regardless of macronutrient adjustment, table Carb1, the idea here is to by eliminating a lot of the sugars and eliminate a lot of the fast foods that we might consume within our diet, we're able to eliminate a lot of the metabolic diseases that are facing us currently, a lot of the overfatness and hyperadiposity that affects us both aesthetically as well as metabolically, as well as in terms of our health.

Table Carb1. Summary of foods allowed, suggested, or not allowed within the ketogenic and paleo diets.

Foods and Food sources permitted	Foods that can be permitted	Foods and food sources forbidden
Animal Meat	Coffee	Cereals and Grains
Animal Fat	Tea	Starchy Fruits
Eggs	No Sugar Sodas	Starchy Vegetables
Fish	High-Lactose Animal-derived milk	Sugary drinks
Low-Lactose Animal-derived milk	High-Lactose Animal-derived dairy	Nut-derived Non-dairy drink
Low-Lactose Animal-derived dairy	Low-glycemic fruits	Nut-derived Non-dairy products
Low-glycemic fruits	Low-glycemic vegetables	High-glycemic legumes
Low-glycemic vegetables	Lower-glycemic legumes	High-sugar alcohol and cocktails
Leafy greens	Soy or Tofu	High-sugar condiments and sauces
Nuts and Seeds	Low-sugar alcoholic beverages	
Nut and Seed oils	Low-sugar "Energy drinks"	
Nut and Seed butters	Low-sugar condiments and sauces	
Nut and Seed flour		

The other thing that needs to be addressed within the guise of the ketogenic diet is the way that we are able to formulate this diet. This is where the low-carbohydrate, the ketogenic diets, and the Atkins diets might differentiate themselves from each other and from the other dietary practices within the trinity of the ketogenic diets.

The first basic principle is that you have to cap your net carbohydrates eaten each day. But what does the net carbohydrate mean? That is the carbohydrates in your diet that are not fiber or a "sugar alcohol" that can be used by the cells of the body as a fuel source for metabolism.

Net Carbs = Total Carbohydrates – Fiber – (Sugar Alcohol + Allulose)

Based on the style of low-carbohydrate diet that is being followed, the cap can be set anywhere from 10 to 15 net grams of carbohydrates per day up to 100 net grams of carbohydrates. With the general premise of the diet dogma being that you will start with 3 to 7-days at the very low end of this net carbohydrate range to serve as an induction to the diet and start the ketogenic shift in your metabolism. It is during this first week of the ketogenic diet that almost everyone will go through what has been called the "Keto Flu" that typically comes from a combination of dehydration and hypoglycemia that is most commonly sensed over the first few days of the beginning of any ketogenic diet. Following the induction and the initiation of the ketogenic metabolism, there is a slow reintroduction of net carbohydrates to the diet over 3 weeks until the upper end of 100 net grams per day has been reached. Along this continuum, there are noted advantages to weight loss on the lower end of the continuum relative to the upper end. In a traditional low-carbohydrate ketogenic diet (Atkins-style diet), the recommendation for food choice is focused on increases in fat consumption while maintaining protein intake to offset loss of Calories from excluding carbohydrates. With carbohydrate sources being either packaged products from the companies or whole foods (i.e., low-glycemic fruits and vegetables) that offer higher fiber content relative to the total carbohydrates.

What do we know about the benefits that get reported for the ketogenic diet?

Well, a lot of it has to do with changes in metabolism based off of changes in our energy utilization, where we're going to change the fuel sources that we're going to follow to get the ATP within the body, where instead of using a lot of carbohydrates, we will predominantly rely on fats for fuel. While we will still use some carbohydrates, the majority of energy metabolism is going to focus on fat utilization throughout most of the activities that we're going to have. By changing from using sugars to using fats, we're going to change a lot of hormone actions that might take place. Some actions that will lead to changes in various types of hormone sensitivity, as well as altering our body compositional ratio (fat mass to fat-free mass). Metabolically and physiologically, we will see distinct changes in the tissues and organ systems of the body while following a ketogenic diet.

Within our adipose tissue, because we're going to change our dietary practices, we're going to end up increasing the utilization of fat and increasing hormone changes that will increase the amount of fat breakdown we might see within adipose tissue. This is going to be accompanied by a change in Insulin sensitivity, a change in hormone signaling, and a change in macrophage signaling from the macrophages from the immune cells that we see within the fat masses of the body. Changes in metabolism at the fat cells are going to lead to changes in hormone signaling coming away from the pancreas, which is going to lead to normalization of Insulin and glucagon, particularly for people who have Insulin and glucagon issues, metabolic issues, due to overfatness. At the liver, we're going to see an increase in gluconeogenesis, the making of glucose from glucose metabolites, as well as an increase in ketone formation due to the restriction that we might have in the total amount of carbohydrates that we're going to consume. What we have to remember is that we need a minimum of 120 grams of carbohydrates each day in order to have the proper amount of glucose for our brain to function appropriately, and at least another 10 grams (or 130 grams each day) for immune and blood cells to function correctly. If we are short in our intake of glucose, then we will have to meet this need for glucose another way, and this is completed by our liver producing more glucose from the glucose metabolites (i.e., pyruvate, lactate, glycerol) circulating around our body through gluconeogenesis.

The change in fat metabolism can also cause an increase in Insulin sensitivity that is going to come about due to changes in normalization of Insulin and glucagon signaling, as well as an increase in ROS clearance due to changes in metabolism is going to reduce the total amount of ROS that we might see within the body due to changes in inflammation. In the nervous system, we're going to see changes in Insulin sensitivity that's going to allow for neuroplasticity and improved neuron function. The changes in Insulin sensitivity, along with a reduction in ROS inflammation damage, have been attributed to the changes that we might see within neurodegenerative diseases for people who follow a ketogenic diet. There is some reported benefit for people who have seizure disorders, where following a ketogenic diet will reduce the total number of seizures and the total level of seizure that might be experienced if one would experience a seizure. Within the musculoskeletal system, we will see various changes in metabolic flexibility; we will change what fuel sources we might use for energy purposes. We will see an increase in Insulin sensitivity, we will see a change in fat mass utilization, fat mass utilization for energy purposes, which means we're going to see an increase in lipolysis and fatty acid oxidation. We may see an increase in protein utilization. However, that increase in protein utilization for energy purposes will be offset by an increase in growth responses, as well as the retention of tissue mass in the bone and skeletal muscle tissue during the weight loss period. In terms of cardiovascular benefit, this is where we see a lot of variability based on how we measure changes within the systems due to the ketogenic diet. With the reduction in inflammation, we may see changes in atherosclerosis and changes in cardiac functions. However, this is not universally seen for everybody following a ketogenic diet based on the ability to metabolize fats within the body.

What costs might a low-carbohydrate diet have?

All of this sounds great, but then we have to think, wait, is it too good to be true? Is it a panacea? Is it something that is going to be a cure-all?

There is some evidence to support that eating keto is not necessarily automatically healthier, and following a high-fat diet may impact my exercise performance, particularly in explosive exercises as well as in long-duration exercises. This second point is interesting given the fact that when we do long-duration exercise or athletic events, we tend to utilize more fat than carbohydrates as our fuel source. But the problem is that changes in fat utilization following a ketogenic diet may lead to a reduction in explosive muscle contraction capability because of the reduction in glycogen and glycogen stores within the muscles.

What else might we have to worry about as it relates to the ketogenic diet... deficiencies? Just like with any other diet that we might follow, if we are not eating what we should be eating, we have to worry about micronutrient deficiencies and macronutrient deficiencies. In this case here, because of the restriction on types of foods that we might be eating, people who follow a ketogenic diet that do not eat large amounts of vegetables, in particular, low glycemic vegetables, may have fiber deficiencies because of the increased use of fat or fuel source; see table Carb2.

Now, a lot of people might say, well, I'm going to be eating large amounts of meat, so why am I going to have an iron deficiency when we know that people who eat animal protein will automatically have higher amounts of iron in their diet relative to people who don't eat animal protein? Because of the foods that we're eating following a ketogenic diet, we may have competition for transport of a lot of these ions. At the same time, because I'm not consuming large amounts of starches and large amounts of sugars, I do not have the ability to absorb a lot of these ions due to current flow across the membranes of the intestine. A lot of the ions that we see listed here are moving with water and water movement. It goes hand in hand, particularly with sodium, as well as with a lot of the starches that we might have, carbohydrates that we might have within our diet, where if I restrict the carbohydrates, I may also restrict the movement of these cations.

Table Carb2. Indication for the potential nutrient deficits following a low-carbohydrate diet (Ketogenic/Atkins, Paleo).

Macronutrient	Minerals	Vitamins and co-factors
Carbohydrates	Iron	Vitamin A
Essential Fatty Acids	Magnesium	Vitamin B_1
Fiber	Potassium	Vitamin B_5
	Selenium	Vitamin B_6
	Sodium	Vitamin B_7
		Vitamin B_9
		Vitamin C
		Vitamin D
		Carnitine

Because of the implicit and explicit good food versus bad food idea, there is a change in psychological drive for foods that may lead to various types of food cravings, but there's also a lot of social exclusion going on within the ketogenic diet. The good food, bad food, and social exclusion lead to a very restrictive diet that can cause social exclusionary behaviors to take place that may limit the likelihood of following the diet for long periods of time. There is a chance that establishing a ketogenic diet can induce a condition known as metabolic acidosis. A condition that is seen when the pH for the body when following the ketogenic diet drops below the range of normal pH (7.35-7.45) that is attributed to the large amount of protein and fat within the diet leading to more acids (i.e., amino acids, fatty acids, ketones) moving in the bloodstream. Speaking of fat, the higher amounts of saturated fat and lower amounts of polyunsaturated fat and monounsaturated fat can lead to cardiovascular issues, especially high blood pressure, if the diet is followed without a combination of exercise. There can also be an imbalance in the ratio between all the saturated fat and monounsaturated fat, as well as the ratio between our omegas, omega-3 and omega-6, which can lead to an altered fat absorption and metabolism taking place within the body. For some people, because of genetic issues, they may have an altered ability to metabolize the cholesterol that's being consumed, which may lead to an increase in LDL levels for individuals who are trying to follow the ketogenic diet.

Along with that, we might also have issues that come about because of the fact that just because I am following a ketogenic diet, we tend to think of the fact that we're following a natural food consumption. Yet, we have to remember that because of popularity, there are a lot of foods that are going to be mass-produced. Additionally, with the intention to reduce sugar but still desiring "sweetness" in our foods and beverages, a lot of times we're going to be consuming non-nutritive sweeteners. Non-nutritive sweeteners and mass-produced processed foods have been shown to have metabolic disruptive characteristics that have been shown to increase the risk for cancer, cardiovascular disease, and disrupt regulation of food intake, body weight issues, and glucose metabolism. Meaning that even though the diet is meant to be used to correct issues of metabolic syndrome and overfatness, the potential presence of metabolic disruptors may interfere with achieving this goal. As consumption of artificial sweeteners, non-nutritive sweeteners have been linked with increased food intake, abnormal Insulin secretions, cardiovascular disease, and abnormal growth signals within skeletal muscles, all mimicking what we might have already seen with people who exhibit metabolic syndrome and overfatness, even though we're consuming these non-nutritive sweeteners in an attempt to reduce caloric intake. Once again indicating that changes in nutrition and changes in diet as they relate to body weight, body composition, and overall health are not about calories. It's about the nutrients that are being consumed. Along with this, non-nutritive sweeteners tend to taste sweeter than normal sugar in terms of their level of sweetness and our bliss point, which may lead to an overconsumption of food in an attempt to get the bliss point of consumption that we are attempting to get from food consumption, which may lead to an increase in nutrient balance towards the consumption side that can lead to an increase in fat mass that we are attempting to combat by following the ketogenic diet.

Paleo Diets

What exactly is a "paleo" diet? The paleo diet is a dietary philosophy that is focused on what we think a Paleolithic human would have eaten for their diet. A dogma that is based on the idea that paleolithic humans were eating a lot of raw or "natural" things such as fish, steak, shellfish, poultry, vegetables, nuts, fruits, berries, and eggs. The idea is that this type of diet is going to counteract a lot of the nutritional deficiencies and health issues that might come about through eating a modern diet with large amounts of fast food and processed foods that lead to a host of metabolic problems and weight issues that impact a majority of individuals today.

What does the evidence say are the benefits?

To begin discussing the benefits and costs of the paleo diet, sometimes referred to as a caveman diet, it is important to remember that most of the recommendations that we are provided from disciples of the paleo diet come from and analysis of modern hunter-gatherer associations and indigenous hunter-gatherer groups, not necessarily what might have been consumed during paleolithic times. We also have to remember that a lot of the foods that we're going to consider to be paleo are actually modern in their derivations, and a lot of foods that we think of as being modern actually were being consumed by our paleolithic relatives. A lot of the benefits that we're going to look at are not universal, and there is some question as to whether or not the benefits that we see coming from diets are coming from the diet or coming from other things.

We do know that there are some benefits that come about from following a paleo, or caveman, dogmatic dietary practice. A lot of these benefits are similar to the benefits that we see coming from things like intermittent fasting, a very low carbohydrate diet, as well as a plant-rich diet. Benefits that include increased Insulin sensitivity and neuroplasticity within the nervous system combined with a reduction in reactive oxidative species damage allow for improvement in the function of neurons that can slow the rate of degeneration and possibly allow for greater amounts of growth to take place under the correct amount of stimulation. There is also an increase in metabolic flexibility, or the ability for cells of the body to use all of the fuel sources when it comes to the energy portion of our metabolism. This shift in fuel use is combined with increased Insulin sensitivity, increase in lipolysis (break down of fats), and an increase in the growth of fat-free tissues within the musculoskeletal system. That, as a result, leads to changes in not only body weight but, more importantly, body composition and is accompanied by changes in fat cell hormones that reduces inflammation responses throughout the body to improve overall health.

There is also noted potential for changes in cardiovascular health, but not universally in a direction of changes that would be deemed beneficial. We do get reports on a change in the blood vessels with a reduction in blood pressure that is associated with reduced atherosclerosis (stiffening of the arteries) and the changes in inflammation and stress hormones. The combination of changes can lead to improvements in heart function and overall heart health. Yet, the change in inflammation is highly questionable in terms of the root cause for the benefit coming from the diet as opposed to other lifestyle changes.

Metabolically, there is an increase in Insulin and Leptin sensitivity that stimulates fat breakdown in the adipose tissues, leading to a reduction in fat mass and a change in hormones coming from fat cell hormones (adipokines) and immune cells that lead to further reduction in inflammation. With changes in metabolism, there is a noted reduction in oxidative stress faced by the body that will also contribute to the reduction in inflammation that we see throughout the body for people who dogmatically follow a Paleolithic diet. As previously noted, we see normalization of Insulin and Leptin responses, but for individuals who have metabolic issues (i.e., type-2 diabetes or metabolic syndrome), there is also a normalization to Glucagon and GLP-1 levels leading to improvement in their overall health. But once again, it is not universal and may be associated with changes in activity as well as other lifestyle interventions. There are also some questionable responses for improvements in our liver. With an increase in sensitivity to Insulin, Glucagon and GLP-1 leading to normalization of glucose metabolism that minimizes the release of glucose from the liver stores or from making new glucose (unless necessary), along with a reduction in oxidative stress and non-alcoholic fatty acid liver syndrome for those who follow a Paleo diet that reduces consumption of refined sugars, non-nutritive sweeteners, and grains. There is also a noted increase in ketone formation due to a change in metabolic functions towards fat utilization and ketogenic processes that can further reduce oxidative stress. Along with the reduced oxidative stress, there is potentially an increase in the clearance of free radicals and oxidative species for people who have metabolic issues and change their diet to follow a Paleo diet.

This sounds great! But what about the entirety of the research? We did say that there were some questionable findings and some responses that were not universally found. And so, the question that comes about is, does it automatically mean a healthier food in our diet?

What are the costs and risks of following this diet?

This is where it becomes important to address the paradox to claims of many dogmatic diets... does eating more unprocessed foods and eating things that are more in line with our ancestral human diets automatically mean a healthier diet? This paradox leads to a problem for a lot of the claims about the ancestral human diet being better, as you have to ignore the evolutionary processes and adaptations that took place throughout our history.

There is also the potential for having nutrient deficiencies because we're going to be cutting out things from the diet, table 2. With the reduction in dairy consumption, we do run the risk of having calcium deficiency as well as vitamin D deficiency. With the reduction in grain consumption, we do risk having B-vitamin deficiencies, in particular the folate, but also with the niacin.

We will also see a change in psychological drive for food more in a Paleo diet than in many of the other diets simply because of the excessive labeling of good food versus bad food. Because of the lower consumption of vegetab es in some of the diets, this is going to be very similar to what we see with a very low-carbohydrate ketogenic diet; we do run the risk of diet-induced metabolic acidosis. The other thing to worry about due to the type of foods that we're eating is an excessive load of animal saturated fat combined with antigens from the food and cholesterol molecules. It is this combination of animal saturated fat and animal antigens that can lead to an actual increase in atherosclerosis, stiffening of the arteries, that might eventually progress to cardiovascular disease. Additionally, those that have genetic mutations that impact their liver's ability to clear cholesterol from the bloodstream are at an increased risk for suffering from hypercholesterolemia (high cholesterol) that not only impacts cardiovascular health but may also impact overall liver functions.

From the Paleo diet, we could not only see large amounts of saturated fats relative to our polyunsaturated fats (PUFAs) and our monounsaturated fats (MUFAs) that can alter fat metabolism and fat absorption taking place, but also altered cholesterol metabolism within the liver, leading to increased levels of circulating LDLs within the body. We should also be concerned about the sources of the PUFAs and MUFAs (i.e., nuts, seeds, grains) that are being eaten, as the paleo diet can disrupt the delicate ratio of omega-6 to omega-3 fatty acids that we consume. Increased consumption of nuts high in omega-6 fatty acids will lead to overconsumption of the omega-6 fatty acids and underconsumption of the omega-3 fatty acids, especially EPA and DHA, that are necessary for proper immune function and hormone production. Deficiencies that might limit any improvements in our overall level of inflammation coming from a paleo diet.

One of the things we have to address within the idea about the Paleo diet is, is it actually truly close to the Paleolithic diet? That is, is it actually historically close to what we would think of as a Paleolithic diet? To answer this question as "yes," we either misapply our historical understanding of dietary practices, or assume that modern hunter-gatherer practices are equivalent to actual Paleolithic dietary practices or fail to include that as we have adapted and evolved, our diets and foods are evolving in tandem. Meaning that for many proponents of the Paleo, or caveman, diet the rationale for why to choose the diet is a misrepresentation of what actually is historically accurate in terms of our dietary practices from 10,000 or 20,000 or 30,000 or even 40,000 years ago. As we were doing a lot of cultivating, doing a lot of agricultural cultivation and domestication taking place, which means a lot of the foods that we think about as being modern aren't actually modern; they're more Paleolithic than we actually attribute in terms of their sourcing. The other thing is, just like with all other diets, we start having mass-produced foods that would be sold as being paleo. Processed foods bring chemical additives into our diet that can and do act like metabolic disruptors, which means that we run the risk of having metabolic disruption taking place from following a Paleo diet. Risks that are very similar to following the modern diets that the paleo advocates preach against, and therefore might limit any of the health benefits that we think about as coming from following this diet. However, if we're to follow a Paleo diet based on the use of meats and vegetables and nuts and berries and fruits without purchasing the mass-produced foods, we may lower the risk of having metabolic disruption depending upon the composition of foods and ratios of nutrients and essential amino acids and fatty acids being consumed.

Carnivore Diet

The ideals and concepts contained within the carnivore diet are a rebirth of the diets first proposed by Cantini and Salisbury in the 1870s and 1880s. The modern version of the carnivore diet has found a new life in the social media feeds across platforms from YouTube to TikTok. With proponents of the carnivore diet presenting it as a nutritional means to somehow cure a whole bunch of various types of health ailments that we might face (e.g., rheumatoid arthritis, diabetes, dementia, cardiovascular disease, irritable bowel syndrome, leaky gut syndrome), along with being a diet that can paradoxically lead to greater amounts of both weight loss and weight gain that is coupled with greater gains in strength.

Proponents of the carnivore diet tend to be the ones reminding us to "drink your protein shakes" while wrapping up a workout, to "let's eat our steak, let's eat our eggs" while disregarding salads, vegetables, fruits, or any of the sugars that might be found in any foods that are not animal protein, table Carb3. Furthering this point to avoid sugars, the disciples will tell everyone to also avoid any of the refined products that we might find within a lot of our diets, even those products found in the other forms of the low-carbohydrate diets. Food products that they attribute as being the cause for health issues that we have seen on the rise throughout our modern time and are generally associated with obesity and overfatness issues.

These proponents of the carnivore diet indicate that not only will the carnivore diet allow for weight loss but it can also let you achieve that weight loss quite rapidly. It will also be a means to maintain weight following weight loss, but also provide the additional protein needed to grow muscle while also encouraging the ability to rebalance our metabolic health.

Table Carb3. Summary of foods and food sources and excluded from diet while following a Carnivore diet.

Foods and Food Sources Allowed	Foods that can be added based on strictness	Foods and Food Sources that are forbidden
Animal Protein Animal Fat Low-Lactose Animal-derived dairy Eggs Fish	Coffee Tea Energy Drinks Nuts Tofu Fiber supplements (no sugar version) Mushrooms Nutritional Yeast	Fruits Vegetables High Lactose Dairy Nut butters and oils Legumes, Nuts, or Seeds Grains and Cereals Processed foods Alcohol and Sugary beverages Honey or Sweeteners

What does science say about the benefits that are being offered?

There appear to be benefits that can arise from the carnivore diet. A lot of the benefits that are attributed to the carnivore diet are coming from the extrapolation of the benefits seen in ketogenic research. That means that most of the benefits that are attributed to the carnivore diet may in fact be coming from the low-carbohydrate diet and not necessarily coming away from the carnivore diet itself. Where it is important to remember that this is but one style of the various styles of low-carbohydrate diets that all tend to offer a similar continuum of health benefits and potential for weight loss. Where the carnivore diet is simply going to an extreme in the low-carbohydrate diet where protein and animal protein in particular will be making up the majority of food and food sources for the diet.

The first benefit that becomes a central discussion point is that there will be weight loss and, in some cases, a rapid weight loss coming from fat mass. At the same time, and paradoxically to this point, proponents will also stipulate that you can gain weight following the exact same dietary practice.

There are also anecdotes of improved mental functions and slowing of dementia or neurodegenerative disease for those that have this metabolic issue. While there might be a reduction in ROS and ROS damage, along with improved Insulin sensitivity and neural growth from a ketogenic and low-carbohydrate diet, there is no direct evidence to support that the carnivore diet by itself will produce benefits beyond what is offered from the ketogenic and low-carbohydrate diets. However, there is a change in food drive that sees greater amounts of satiety, feeling full, for longer periods of time by utilizing a carnivore-style diet. Changes in feeding and hunger that can lead to less total nutrient consumption that gets combined with limited to no carbohydrates in the diet that shifts metabolism to break down tissues (primarily fat) of the body to meet nutrient needs and the resultant weight loss that is being sought. The result of which is the reduction in fat mass and possible total body weight that proponents of the diet claim to be a principal benefit.

As with the other low-carbohydrate diets, we see an increase in metabolic flexibility. Accompanying these changes in metabolism, there is a general reduction in some inflammatory signals and chronic inflammation that has been seen in those that are highly sedentary or exhibited overfatness issues prior to starting a higher-protein, low-carbohydrate diet. Changes that stem from modification in the metabolic functions in the adipose (fat) cells and the hormones being produced that change immune cell signaling that can lead to reduction in inflammation and improve metabolic functions throughout the body. A change that sees an increase in Insulin and Leptin sensitivity, normalization of hormones related to regulating glucose levels in the blood (i.e., Insulin, Glucagon, Cortisol, Epinephrine, GLP-1), matched by an increase in breakdown of fats to be used for fuel. These responses lead to a rationale for why we can see rapid changes in diabetic indices for people who are prediabetic or who have been diagnosed with type-2 diabetes when using this dogmatic diet.

The changes seen in fat breakdown and modification in fat cell metabolism are the greatest metabolic changes seen related to the weight loss coming from the carnivore diet. The impact of the changes in metabolic flexibility will be met with maintenance of bone and skeletal muscle mass when following a carnivore diet for weight loss, while it may also increase growth of muscle and bone when combined with resistance exercise and resistance training. There will also be changes in liver functions that can be beneficial. The reduction in carbohydrate load might change fatty-acid deposition, and changes in ROS-induced damage can reduce or resolve non-alcoholic fatty-acid liver syndrome. The modification in hormones related to glucose regulation impacts both the non-alcoholic fatty-acid issues and the rate of gluconeogenesis through changes in GLP-1 and Insulin sensitivity antagonistically acting on the actions of Glucagon.

There is indication that for those with irritable bowel syndrome or suffering from "leaky" gut syndrome, a switch to a carnivore diet can improve symptoms. The improvement is associated with a reduction of immune cell activation within the intestines along with a reduction in the overall rate of movement of materials through the intestines during the digestion and absorption of the meals that are being consumed.

What are the costs and risks of using the carnivore diet?

So, carnivore diets can adversely impact liver function through an increase in transamination and deamination reactions along with increases in urea and ammonia formation due to the increase in amino acid metabolism and protein breakdown taking place within the liver so as to meet energetic requirements in fuel source. Production of urea and ammonia can contribute to an increased risk for gout for those that follow a carnivore diet for a longer duration. It appears that a carnivore diet can impact liver enzyme functions and liver enzyme activities in the long term, even if it can resolve issues surrounding non-alcoholic fatty acid liver issues. Impairment of enzyme actions can have an adverse impact on detoxification reactions and cholesterol metabolism in the liver. And can subsequently impact metabolic activity throughout the body.

Metabolically, there is an increased chance for having metabolic acidosis. Acidosis that occurs from the dietary restrictions leading to an increased rate of ketone formation and circulation of amino acids and fatty-acids. Additionally, there can be a negative impact on liver functions and lipoprotein metabolism that can lead to greater amounts of triglycerides, LDL and total cholesterol, with limited change in HDL. Alterations in fat and cholesterol metabolism can have an impact on the transportation of fat-soluble vitamins around the body. It is the altered fat and cholesterol metabolism and fat absorption that can lead to an increase in blood lipid profiles and why we cannot necessarily state that a carnivore diet leads to a reduction in blood lipids or cholesterol relative to somebody who's following a simple ketogenic diet or other dietary dogmatic practices.

There's no direct evidence, although there are a lot of anecdotes, that the diet provides benefits to cardiovascular health. There is a change in lipid metabolism that might allow for a degree of improvement, but with increased animal fat consumption. There is also a change of fats being deposited within the cardiac muscle of the heart. A change that can lead to an increase in fat droplets (i.e., triglycerides) in the cardiac muscle and lead to greater adipose tissue around the heart that adversely impacts overall heart health. There can also be adverse effects on cholesterol levels and triglycerides in the blood that might increase atherosclerosis (stiffening of the arteries) and result in poor blood vessel function and higher blood pressure that will also adversely impact heart function, reducing heart health.

As with other dogmatic dietary practices, we have to worry about nutrient deficits. While there is some indication based on one author's review article to indicate nutrients in the foods allowed by the carnivore diet can meet our nutrient needs, this might be compromised based on the strictness of dogmatic adherence and selection of foods. With greater adherence and more restrictive choices for the source of protein, nutrient deficiencies can arise. The deficits coming from the carnivore diets are not solely from the types of foods being eaten or avoided but also due to the diet's impact on metabolism that is similar to what we see from the other low-carbohydrate diets, table Carb4.

Table Carb4. Potential nutrient deficiencies that can arise from following the carnivore diet. # indicates potential deficiency based on food source and quality of animal protein, *Indicates potential deficiency due to metabolic use not from food.

Macronutrient	Mineral	Vitamin and co-factors
Anti-oxidants	Calcium	Vitamin B_6
Fiber	Chloride	Vitamin B_7
Carbohydrates	Iron	Vitamin C
Essential Fatty-acids	Iodine	Vitamin D #*
Polyunsaturated Fatty-acids	Magnesium	Vitamin E
Monounsaturated Fatty-acids	Potassium	Vitamin K #
	Selenium	Carnitine*
	Sodium	Flavonoids

It is the macronutrient deficiencies that cause the rapid weight loss from the carnivore diet, yet the dietary-induced deficiencies and potential metabolic issues that can arise mean that even though one might seek out a pathway for weight loss, it potentially is an unhealthy way to achieve that loss. Based on foods consumed, we develop deficits in carbohydrates that are necessary in order to maintain gastrointestinal health (e.g., fiber), or the carbohydrates and ions to maintain normal metabolic functions (e.g., glucose, omega-3 fatty acids, sodium, iodine). The limited intake of carbohydrates means an overreliance on gluconeogenesis to meet the glucose needs along with depletion of glycogen stores that can impact the performance of skeletal muscle during athletic activities or during prolonged higher-intensity exercise. Based on metabolic actions, we might have deficits in vitamins and metabolic cofactors (e.g., B vitamins, vitamin D, carnitine) that can impact the ability to use fats for fuel by the cells of the body or regulate oxidative stresses.

The regulation of eating and the psychological drive for food can also cause adverse eating behaviors and responses based on the idea of good and bad foods that should be in your diet. An issue that can make a carnivore diet exceedingly onerous to follow given the restriction to what can and cannot be consumed if the diet is not a self-selected pattern of eating. Additionally, the carnivore diet can lead to hypoglycemia and an increase in signals (i.e., metabolite depletion, regulatory hormones) that trigger hunger in excess. Excess hunger is known to lead to overeating and is coupled with an attempt to eat enough food to receive the bliss response from the reward center of the brain. A response that typically comes from sensing foods that are pleasurable to eat (based on a combination of senses) that might be available from eating large portions of meat with limited "sweet" or "umami" foods. The overconsumption of proteins can have a secondary side effect, excessive digestive thermal effect, i.e., the meat sweats.

A carnivore diet can adversely impact gastrointestinal functions; ever with the indication for relieving issues such as irritable bowel issues, the very low-fiber and residual fiber in the diet not only impact digestive functions but can also impact our microbiome. Changes in the microbiome coupled with high amounts of animal fat and animal antigens, increased saturated fat consumption relative to unsaturated fat, and an imbalance in the omega-6 to omega-3 ratio can lead to a state of inflammation along with impacting the ability to form inflammatory hormones and normal fat metabolism within the cells of the body.

One of the rationales given to avoid a carnivore diet is the impact that high-protein diets have on kidney functions. However, this antiquated idea that having a high-protein diet would lead to kidney issues and chronic kidney disease is not supported. While this is true for anyone with a history of kidney disease, there is limited evidence to support everyone having altered kidney function following a high-protein diet. The advice that is necessary and leads to the last of the limitations and deficiencies that might occur is that there needs to be excess in fluid consumption to maintain being normally hydrated.

What can be said about the low-carbohydrate diets: the ketogenic, paleo, and carnivore diets?

The use of diets that minimize sugar intake has become very popular in the last few years, especially with the view that any added sugar is dangerous. While there are a variety of methods to follow in the low-carbohydrate dogmatic approaches, each with the intention that by reducing the overall intake of carbohydrate, you are able to reverse metabolic health issues and, as a benefit, lose body weight. Improvements that stem from the belief that following a diet that reduces glucose levels that lowers Insulin and by lowering Insulin the body will reduce fat being stored and improve cardiometabolic function independent of any actual weight loss.

Pros

- Improved metabolic health: increased metabolic flexibility coupled with improved glucose regulation and Insulin, Leptin, Glucagon, GLP-1 sensitivity, and reduced inflammation signals
- Improved cardiovascular fitness: when appropriately followed, there can be reduced LDL levels and vessel inflammation leads to better blood pressure and overall heart functions
- Weight loss with retention of fat-free mass: change in fat metabolism leads to reduced fat mass and total body weight, with higher protein intake limits the loss of fat-free mass during weight loss
- Resolution of intestinal immune issues: reduced inflammation responses and allergen exposure in intestines reduce "leaky gut" and irritable bowel syndromes along with issues associated with Crohn's and celiac that can be triggered by gluten exposure

Cons

- The diet can be complex and restrictive: you need to determine balance points for Calories and nutrient loads and then changes in those balance points based on carbohydrate loads. The dietary premise restricts what is and what is not eaten based on foods that can make it feel excessively onerous, and this can limit the likelihood for long-term follow through

- Negative impact on neuron functions, exercise, or athletic performance: limited glucose and carbohydrates in the diet can impact how well neurons function (primary fuel source is glucose) and minimize the explosive muscle contractions that are needed during exercise and athletic events.
- Potential of liver issues: the increase in fat and cholesterol can alter liver fat and cholesterol metabolism; with higher protein intake, there is an increased stress that can be placed on the liver to complete transamination and deamination of amino acids.
- Potential for gout: increased amino acid metabolism at the liver leads to greater production of ammonia and urea that can lead to gout issues.
- Potential for gastrointestinal issues: the higher fat and protein, and lower fiber in the diet increases the risks for gallbladder and pancreatic issues and for constipation
- Potential for dehydration: because of the low carbohydrate load, there is a potential to become dehydrated that must be met with increased fluid and electrolyte consumption

Take-home message:

Lower carbohydrate diets can be safe and effective, with ample evidence to support their use for body compositional change, and improvement in metabolic health and cardiovascular disease. Tenets of these diets are becoming more mainstream across various dogmatic practices, with the advice to look at sugars in the food we buy stemming from the general premise of this dogmatic diet. Even though the application has flaws outside of people that might have metabolic syndrome or are suffering effects of overfatness, the awareness of nutrients in food is a positive takeaway from a low-carbohydrate diet. What needs to be reinforced is that even though there are anecdotes of performance benefits, there is little evidence to show improvements in cognitive functions or athletic performance.

Old MacDonald had a farm...

*"Old MacDonald had a farm, E-I-E-I-O
And on that farm he had a pig, E-I-E-I-O
With a oink-oink here and a oink-oink there
Here a oink, there a oink, everywhere a oink-oink..."*

Of the dogmatic diets that have come into vogue since the turn of the century, none has taken hold as fast and as prevalent as the perception that organic food is healthier and more nutritious for a person. A premise that is cultivated in a diet dogma that has its roots in this organic movement, farm-to-table or eating locally grown and locally sourced foods. But where did this movement start, and why has it become so entrenched in the dogmatic discussions that we have around food.

The idea of organic farming is nothing new in the sense of a modern phenomenon. The idea of farming throughout human history, until the development of synthetic fertilizers, herbicides, and pesticides, is what one might deem to be an organic perspective. With the growing use of these substances to increase crop yield, there came a movement as a way to get farming "back to its root" of relying on natural systems that plants offer to allow them to grow and protect themselves from insects or from other plants that might compete for nutrients from the soil.

While both locally sourced foods and the use of organic gardening on a mass-marketed scope have their roots in the 1940s, they really took hold in the 1960s and 1970s with the growth of farmer co-ops and markets. The movement grew in popularity based on the premise that comes from the hallmark of the three primary promises that proponents advocate whenever discussing organic and locally sourced foods. First, it takes food and agriculture back to their evolutionary historical basis, and based on nutrition tenets, organic and locally sourced food is inherently healthier for you. Second, organic farming and locally sourced foods will contribute to having sustainable food in the market with growing importance on the international stage as a way to reduce the tax that agriculture has on the environment, causing less pollution, slowing soil loss, and increasing local biodiversity. And lastly, it reinforces local communities and economies by keeping money within the community, as opposed to sending it to multinational corporations that are typically found throughout agribusiness, even if the organic sector of groceries accounts for hundreds of billions of dollars each year and includes many multinational companies having products in the organic food marketplace.

So, what makes up the diet of an organic and locally sourced diet?

It is important to understand that marketing and designation of organic is not based on scientific standards but is assigned based on a checklist from regulator standards, i.e., USDA Agricultural Marketing or EU Organic certification. To achieve this designation, food producers must not grow plants from genetically engineered (GMO) seeds and must be grown without the use of synthetic (artificial) pesticides, herbicides, or fertilizers. Animals must be raised on feed that does not contain antibiotics and with minimal use of additive hormones to promote growth. For both meat and produce, there need to be minimal chemical preservatives, and seeds should not have been irradiated prior to planting. A secondary characteristic of organic farming is the urging for farmers to actively promote land preservation and livestock treated humanely. Extending this to the locally sourced food, the labeling is an indication that food travels no more than 250 miles from farm or factory to store or restaurant.

Unlike many of the other dogmatic diets that label "good" foods and "bad" foods based on the macronutrients being included or excluded in the diet, the ideal of the organic diet is about the way that the food itself is grown or produced. One of the ways that we see organic foods discussed is as food that is more natural, or as being natural food. The premise that comes from the conjecture of using natural to describe organic foods is that any food that does not get identified as organic is somehow unnatural. This is where a lot of the most boisterous proponents for the diet voice the idea of needing to be able to pronounce ingredients found in food in order to be a food worth eating, a healthy food.

Stemming from this idea about needing to be able to know the words in the ingredients comes the idea that organic foods, or those thought to be natural, are seen as being "chemical free" and are marketed as such, even if this is scientifically an impossibility. There is also the thought that organic foods are toxin-free and intrinsically better than foods that are deemed conventionally farmed. An idea that is coupled with the notion that the foods have greater nutritional density and higher concentrations of micronutrients relative to the conventionally farmed counterparts.

There is also the misguided notion that organic diets are safer as they eliminate or avoid eating any genetically engineered foods (GMO). A thought based on the premise is that these foods become unsafe because of the manipulation of the organisms genes through the insertion of selective and beneficial genes from a different species. A process that proponents of organic diets states makes the produce, or meat, somehow synthetic or artificial and where consumption of such materials might alter one's own metabolic processes. A position that is not supported in any way. Given that all foods are digested and absorbed following digestion in the same manner, the body would not care about the source (i.e., organic or GMO) of the foods being eaten. Ideals about eating and including or excluding foods lead to the obvious question..

What does science say about organic foods and following an organic or locally sourced diet?

The reasons consumers are increasingly choosing organic over conventional food products are varied, including many reasons besides personal health and well-being, such as environmental concerns or animal welfare impact. However, the major determinant behind consumer purchases of organic products is the belief that organic food is healthier or has a superior nutritional profile. Yet, those that tend to follow an organic diet also tend to have a higher ratio of plant to animal foods in their diet. There is also a strong relationship between vegetarian or vegan dogmatic practices within the followers of the tenets of the organic dietary practice. A general trend in food consumption that also follows a tenet that increases whole foods over processed foods, minimizes the consumption of ultra-processed foods (outside of those that have been deemed to be "organic" and align with the premise of what the individual chooses to eat) and becomes highly restrictive in the consumption of processed organic foods containing chemical additives. Meaning that there could be confounds in any conclusions that might be drawn from research examining the health benefits that might arise from consuming organic foods.

The notion that organic food may be healthier has some support. Most of the support stems from the limited use of pesticides and herbicides, i.e., glyphosates, organophosphates (that have been associated with disrupting metabolism and increasing the risk for cancer), in the growing of produce, leading to lower residual levels of these compounds in organic produce. A reduction that leads to lower potential for metabolic disruption that glyphosates and organophosphates might have on overall metabolic function. There is also the reduction in preservatives and non-nutritive sweeteners and high-fructose syrups that limit endocrine and metabolic disruption coming from foods that are being consumed.

While the proponents talk about food being more nutritious, there appears to be little variation between organic and conventional food products, Table Organic1, in terms of macronutrient (e.g., protein, fat, carbohydrate, and dietary fiber) values. There is some evidence to support small differences in the amount of selective macronutrient levels (e.g., omega-3 fatty acids) in organic meats due to feed differences relative to the conventionally farmed livestock. There are similar minor differences in micronutrient composition relative to a conventional diet or a proportionality diet that is recommended by government and health agencies (see *Calories go in… Calories go out*). However, even with differences noted in nutrients, there is no indication that the quantity or bioavailability would lead to a metabolic difference that would favor organic produce or meat when compared to conventionally farmed produce or meat.

Table Organic1. Differences favoring the use of an organic food diet for nutrient availability between organic and conventionally farmed produce and meat.

Macronutrient, Vitamin and coenzyme	Minerals
Omega-3 fatty acid Vitamin C Anthocyanins Flavonoids Carotenoids Lutein Polyphenol antioxidants	Iron Magnesium Phosphorus Potassium

There is speculation that bacteria and pathogens are lower in organic meats, yet there is no evidence to support this speculation. This speculation carries over to the antibiotic resistance in bacteria-contaminated meats, yet there is once again limited evidence to support this speculation and it predominantly stems from the idea that since animals are not being fed animal feed containing antibiotics, then the risk for antibiotic resistance is lessened. A speculation that is excessively complex and fundamentally flawed. There are also reports of lower levels of heavy metals (i.e., cadmium) in organically grown grains but not in fruits or vegetables relative to the conventionally grown produce, yet levels in these metals are extremely low in conventional farming practices and tend to not lead to any adverse issues.

There is speculation that by eating meat and consuming dairy that has not been given additional hormones, the products are somehow inherently safer. These are not true or justified statements. Hormones are present in all living organisms that we eat. In the plants and the animals, and even fungi that make up our diets. The hormones that proponents of the organic diet dogma preach against have an excessively low half-life, and the amount of hormone that may be added to benefit the animals used for milking or for meat is miniscule. Additionally, in order to have an impact on our metabolism and overall health, we would need to be exposed to that hormone in a dose and over a duration that cannot be seen from the products that organic dogmatics preach against.

What benefits might arise from following an organic diet?

The benefits that we see from the organic diet dogma are limited, and many claims that are offered are scientifically dubious. However, evidence that we do have points to lower residue to organophosphates and glyphosates in produce that is farmed following organic practices. Reduced residue may limit the metabolic disruption and potentially carcinogenic effects that the pesticides and herbicides have on our body. There is potential to have higher levels of antioxidants in the diet using an organic dietary practice; however, the higher amounts of antioxidants can be a double-edged sword and could potentially cause more harm than good (see Superfoods in *I need a remedy*).

The consumption of locally sourced foods has the potential to have a positive environmental impact on greenhouse emission given the shorter travel distance that foods have between the source of production and the site of consumption. The ideal that farming using an organic method is more sustainable and humane is hypothetically true; however, the evidence that we have may not support this contention. Yet, the lower rates of nitrites and nitrates being spread over vast acres of land may provide a positive environmental impact, should organic processes expand at a high enough rate to counter the large farming practices utilized by the agribusiness conglomerates. Additionally, the use of crop rotations, a once common practice, can lead to better land management and control of erosion of farmland.

What are the costs or risks of following an organic diet?

As with many of the trendy dietary dogmas, the use of mass-produced and processed foods becomes integral to the foods included in the diet. With greater consumption of processed foods comes potential exposure to metabolic disruptors that can contribute to metabolic issues and overfatness health issues for those that follow the organic dogmas. Additionally, with increased consumption of plant-based foods comes increased exposure to anti-nutrients that can impact digestion and absorption of nutrients along with the ability to use various minerals and electrolytes in metabolic processes taking place in the cells and tissues of the body.

Environmentally, there may be a greater environmental tax on watersheds and aquifers, especially for crops that are high water consumers that do not employ genetically engineered methods (GMO) to reduce water dependency. There is also the potential to spread bacterial contamination through the use of manure and animal waste as fertilizers.

What can we say about the organic diet and eating locally sourced foods?

Organic foods and following organic diet dogmas have been contentious topics. Many followers of this dogmatic diet have argued that organic foods are healthier for you and for the environment relative to their non-organic or conventional food counterparts. However, the differences between these two options are more complicated than they may seem.

Pros

- Potentially higher levels of micronutrients and omega-3 essential fatty acids relative to conventionally farmed foods
- Potentially reduced exposure to pesticide and herbicide residue on produce
- Potentially lower environmental impact
- Potentially fresher produce and non-frozen meat products when purchasing locally sourced
- Potential economic impact by allowing for money to flow and stay locally, supporting local farmers

Cons

- Costs and restrictiveness in food selection and options. Because of the trendiness of having products being labeled as "organic," the cost to the consumer will be higher than purchasing a non-organic or conventional counterpart. A price that is paid even when the products being sold as "organic" may not actually be organic.
- Socially restrictive because of the cost, the ability to find organic options (even with the trendiness) in restaurants outside of niche options can be very limited, and locally sourced or farm-to-table tends to be seasonally restricted, meaning that socialization around meals can be restricted.
- Misinformation and disinformation campaigns lead to misleading and dangerous dietary information being propagated. Many followers of the organic diet dogmas preach that one needs to be able to read and understand the words in the ingredient lists with the implication of such statements that use scientific terminology, which automatically means the foods are less healthy or more dangerous, along with the impetus that one needs to eat "chemically free," something that is

impossible given that everything is made of chemicals and our body needs chemicals in order to perform the metabolism required for life.

- Possible increased risk of exposure to pesticide, herbicide, and fertilizer residues. The idea that the uses of "natural" pesticides, or herbicides automatically means "safer" or "harmless" is misleading, it's important to note that "natural" doesn't automatically mean "harmless," and organic farming still requires pesticides and herbicides that can expose someone to residues that can act as metabolic and endocrine disruptors similar to the synthetic chemicals used in conventional farming methods.

- Possible increased risk of exposure to pathogens through the use of manure and animal waste in fertilizers. Similar to the herbicides and pesticides, simply being "natural" does not automatically mean "safer" or "harmless." The use of manure and animal waste can transfer pathogens and microbes onto produce that can lead to infections from eating produce that has not been thoroughly cleaned or cooked to appropriate temperatures.

Take-home message

The idea of organic food and forming an organic diet is based on the general premise that eating organic is healthier for you and better for the planet. And eating locally sourced foods is better for the environment and local economies by reducing greenhouse gas emissions needed to transport food while keeping money circulating within the local community by supporting local farmers. Yet, the process that leads to what is deemed to be organic versus conventional is both confusing and lacking in scientific consensus about these general ideals.

In terms of nutrition, organic and conventional foods are about evenly matched, while the claims about being environmentally friendly may not be true given the scale of farming necessary to meet demands may make organic farming not entirely an environmentally sustainable approach. Additionally, the cost of following this diet dogma makes it a restricted dietary practice that is often seen by outsiders to be practiced by self-absorbed and snobbish people who are able to afford the costlier foods. As companies have found through marketing and market share, having products indicated as being organic increases profit by allowing you to charge more for the organically labeled products versus a product indicated as being non-organic or conventionally grown. Expenses that are passed along under the guise that someone is buying foods that are somehow better for them to eat. Yet, we lack the scientific consensus on how true that premise is and whether the organic products are really worth the extra costs. With increases in the availability of "organic" products, there comes a question that must be addressed; can mass-marketed products actually be grown, raised, and produced at the escalating rates that we see in the stores, given that less than 8% of farmland in the United States and 12% globally are deemed to follow organic standards? A question that leads to much of the confusion regarding organic diet dogmas is that we can have foods with different designations of "organic" that get lost with all other labeling presented to a consumer.

Everywhere you go,
there we are...

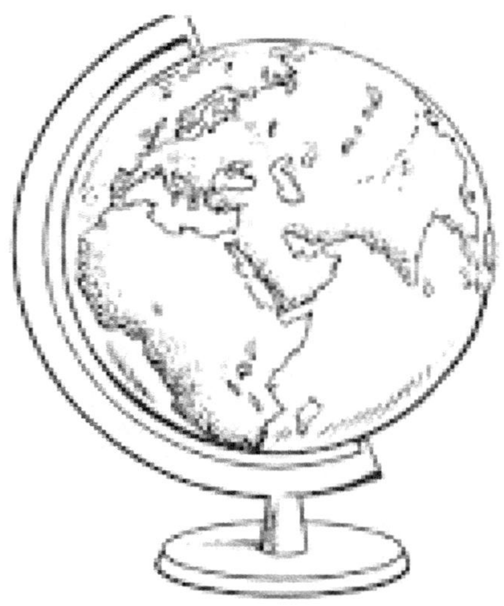

Of the diets that have become dogmatically followed, none has had the historical rise through the media quite like the Mediterranean diet. Not only has the Mediterranean diet become popular to discuss in the media and press, but it has also become integrated into the lexicon of many of the medical diets (see *I need a remedy*). At the same time, it is not the only dietary practice that can be seen as a location-based or region-based dietary dogma. I know, this is where you automatically go with the thought of the **South Beach Diet** as a location-based diet, but **South Beach Diet** is really just a marketing name for a diet that mirrors the low-carbohydrate or ketogenic diet and is not really a region-based diet. Even though the idea is that it originated in South Beach, Miami, FL, USA, which it most likely did not.

Hallmarks of location-based or region-based diet dogma is a diet that is based and focused on ethnic or regional foods that are fundamental to that area's culture. Even though there is a degree of societal impact on dietary restrictions and inclusions that can mirror what gets seen in religious restrictions on foods in the diet, these are not religious diets. This idea can be seen through the marketing and advertisement regarding specific foods or means of preparing food, Table Local1, even those deemed to be the *unhealthy* "Western" or American diets that typically gets linked with the fast-food companies that span the globe.

Table Local1. Examples of diets that originate from specific cultures that can lead to dogmatic dietary practice, including religious diets.

Ahimsa (Hindu, Buddhism, Sikhism)	Kosher
Buddhism	Latter Day Saints (Mormonism)
Cajun	Mediterranean
East Asian	Nordic
Halal	Rastafarian
Indigenous People's (American, Australian, African)	Seventh Day Adventists
	Traditional Polynesian

Mediterranean Diet

To begin our discussion here, we will specifically view the Mediterranean diet. The term and idea of the Mediterranean diet stem from dietary practices first put forth by Ancel Keys in his public health push to reduce the amount of animal-based fat and fat in general from the American diet in the 1960s. Yet, when it comes to foods that are included or cooking methods that are incorporated into this dietary dogma, it is important to realize and note that there is no single definition of a Mediterranean diet. The difficulty comes from the diversity of dietary habits of the 20-plus countries that reside along the

Mediterranean Sea, each with slightly different dietary practices and dogmas. Yet, we are drawn to what Ansel Keys concluded about the food and traditional eating patterns found in the coastal area of Napoli (Italy) in the late 1950s and early 1960s as the definition given for foods and food preparation would be deemed "Mediterranean" in our dogmatic practices of eating. Yet, recent modifications to the ideals have added to what Keys saw as the traditional Napoli diet to include foods and cooking methods from Greece, Crete, and even the French Riviera and Southern Spain.

Table Local2A. Examples of Plant-based Foods that are included as being accepted as part of the Mediterranean diet.

Grains and Legumes	Seeds, Nuts, and Spices	Fruits	Vegetables
Barley	Almonds	Apples	Artichokes
Beans (Cannellini,	Pine Nuts	Apricots	Arugula
Chickpeas, Fava,	Pistachios	Avocado	Beets
Green, Kidney,	Walnuts	Berries	Bell Peppers
Navy)	Anise	Cherries	Broccoli
Buckwheat	Basil	Citrus (Clementines,	Bulbs (Onions,
Bulgur wheat	Bay leaves	Grapefruits, Lemons,	Garlic, Scallions,
Couscous	Chili Pepper	Oranges, Tangerines)	Shallots)
Farro	Cinnamon	Cucumber	Cabbage
Lentils	Clove	Eggplants	Carrots
Oats	Cumin	Grapes	Celery
Orzo	Dill weed	Melons (Honeydew,	Greens
Peas (Split,	Mint	Cantaloupe,	(Dandelion,
Yellow)	Nutmeg	Watermelon)	Mustard)
Quinoa	Oregano	Okra	Kale
Wheat berries	Paprika	Olives	Leeks
	Parsley	Pears	Potatoes
	Rosemary	Pomegranates	Radishes and
	Sage	Stone Fruits (Dates,	Turnips
	Sesame seeds	Figs, Nectarines,	Spinach
	Sumac	Peaches)	Tomatoes
	Tahini	Squashes (Pumpkin,	
	Thyme	Squash, Zucchini)	

Table Local2B. Examples of Animal-derived foods, meats and meat substitutes that are included as being accepted as part of the Mediterranean diet.

Meats	Animal-derived products	Meat Substitutes
Fish (Salmon, Sardine, Tuna) Fowl (chicken, duck, geese, wild game) Meat (Beef, Goat, Lamb, Pork) Seafood and Shellfish (Octopi, Squid, Shrimp, Crab)	Cheese (Brie, Feta, Goat cheeses, Halloumi, Manchego, Parmigiano, Pecorino, Ricotta) Eggs Milk (Cow, Goat) Yogurt (Greek)	Mushrooms Tofu

If we were to develop a "traditional Mediterranean diet" for ourselves based on the characteristics first listed by Keys, it would be characterized as having a proportionality diet based on servings per day mixed with the tenets of a plant-based diet. With the focus on food and food groups for us to eat larger portions of grains, fruits, and vegetables with minimal to no consumption of refined and processed foods and sweets; Tables Local2A and Local2B. While we might expect to see restrictions on meats and animal-derived products, there is actually no real restriction to eating meat or the type of meat that one might choose to eat as long as the amount of high-fat animal meat (e.g., red meat) is limited, but no restriction is seen for equally fatty fish or dairy cheeses (even when kept in "moderation") in the diet. The one real dietary restriction here is to focus dietary fat on the "good" versus "bad" fats that might be seen in the diet with the emphasis on limiting animal-derived saturated fats while consuming higher amounts of omega-3 and omega-6 fatty acids.

There is also what appears to be a requisite consumption of alcohol, especially red wine, in the diet along with ample use of vinegars (e.g., apple cider, wine) as condiments. Paradoxically to many other "healthy" diets, there is no limit to oil use; however, the oil that is most regularly integrated into the diet appears to be the olive oil. The focus on olive oil in the Mediterranean diet and the subsequent indication of the health benefits of the diet and, by extension olive oil, may explain the growing popularity of olive oil in home cooking over the last few decades.

It is the popularity of the diet along with the flexibility offered in food choices that leads to its application across multiple medical dietary practices (see *I need a remedy*) but also the modification of the diet to meet different socioeconomic or ethnocentric standards. Modifications that have led to applications of the Mediterranean diet for diabetics, as a low-carbohydrate or ketogenic diet, as being applied in the context of indigenous dietary practices or in combination with a "Western" or American dietary practice.

The adaptability of the diet across the gambit of health issues we face and cultures around the globe leads to the obvious question.

What does the science say about the claims of benefits coming from a Mediterranean diet?

This is where any quick search of the internet provides millions of returns, all listing hundreds of potential benefits from the Mediterranean diet and claims of being subjectively the "best" diet that it appears we should be discussing as the Superfood of all Superfoods (see *I need a remedy*) and not as a diet. Here is just a smattering of purported benefits that advocates claim come from following the Mediterranean diet: improve cholesterol and lower blood pressure, better cognitive and brain function, reduce episodes of anxiety and/or depression, reduce health issues of overfatness and risk for non-communicable diseases (i.e., metabolic syndrome, heart disease, cancer, neuropathy), reduce severity of autoimmune issues (e.g., lupus, eczema, rheumatoid arthritis), improve digestive functions, reduce oxidative stress and ROS damage, improve weight control and weight loss.

Of this list touting the benefits from the diet, we have evidence to support improvements in cardiometabolic health and blood pressures that is linked with a reduction in cholesterol levels, especially the "harmful" low-density lipoprotein (LDL). The rationale offered for these findings is linked with an increase in antioxidant consumption, reduction in saturated fats, and metabolic disruptors that reduce oxidative stress and issues associated with chronic inflammation, coming from either or both metabolic disruptors and oxidative stress.

The change in metabolic health is associated with changes in glucose metabolism and hormones associated with glucose metabolism, namely Insulin. Changes that lead to improvement in Insulin sensitivity that, when coupled with changes in total carbohydrate load, lead to changes in fat metabolism that further improve cardiometabolic health, leading to improvement in sensitivity to Insulin, Leptin, Ghrelin, GLP-1, and other hormones associated with overall metabolic rates. Along with changes in metabolism and inflammation, there are noted changes in Insulin sensitivity and oxidative stress in the neurons of the brain that slow any degenerative changes that might have started and might even assist with neuron growth and adaptations, allowing for improved cognition, memory, and mood regulation.

Along with improvements in cardiometabolic health, when combined with increased physical activity and exercise or restriction in nutrient consumption (as incorrectly measured by Calories), the Mediterranean diet is linked with weight loss. However, this change is universal for all who have tried the diet, nor does it appear to allow for long-term weight modification.

What are the costs and risks of following a Mediterranean diet?

The ability to answer this question is tricky. The abundance of research that we have has been consistently positive with benefits upon benefits upon benefits being touted; one might be left to conclude that there are no costs or risks to following the Mediterranean diet. Yet, this is not entirely the case when we delve into the potential mechanism being offered for why all the benefits are occurring.

The first issue that must be addressed is the lack of appreciation of genealogical heritage and lifestyle in the application of the Mediterranean diet. This lack of appreciation means that we tend to neglect genetic influence on metabolic responses that can be seen in response to changing diets to match the generalized Mediterranean diets. Influences that might explain why those consuming high amounts of antioxidants may not have adverse effects from excessive antioxidant consumption. A point that must be made given that the primary claim of benefit comes from the "antioxidant" rich foods that are found in the diet. While antioxidants are important, the consumption of foods containing antioxidants needs to be Baby Bear, that is being just right. Increased consumption of antioxidants independent of elevated oxidative stress, such as what is seen with compromised cardiometabolic health, can actually lead to the oxidative stress that they are meant to neutralize. The other aspect being ignored is the general lifestyle that is followed by the people that the diet was modeled after, a population that is generally more active and less sedentary. An important point that is erroneously ignored, given the importance that physical activity has on the factors that the proponents of the diet stipulate as coming from the diet. In fact, if we were to view the importance of factors in developing overall health, physical activity and exercise may be more important than any individual component of a diet.

The other factor that tends to get lost in the translation about using the Mediterranean diet comes into how the diet gets applied. The evidence that we have based on adherence to the diet benefits comes from the totality of change and not from changes in individual foods or food choices from the litany of foods that make up the diet. Meaning that simply adding nuts or using olive oil in lieu of other oil options does not lead to improvements in cardiometabolic health or provide the basis for losing weight. Along the same lines as this issue comes the risk that might arise from increased consumption of nuts, fish, and vegetables in the diet, which is the greater intake of omega-6 fatty acids relative to the omega-3 fatty acids that might lead to inflammatory responses instead of anti-inflammatory responses that are being sought. This gets coupled with the potential increase in consumption of the anti-nutrient compounds that might interfere with digestion and absorption of nutrients in the food or use of the nutrients at the cells and tissues of the body.

What can we say about the Mediterranean Diet?

There are a host of potential and possible benefits that might arise from following the Mediterranean diet, yet the diet needs to be seen in the context of the larger lifestyle of those individuals who served as the basis for the diet's invention. An idea that needs to be extended to almost all dietary interventions that claim the diet leads to improvements in overall health and possibly body composition or body weight. As we know, overall health is a highly complex interaction of several factors (e.g., physiological, psychological, and cultural/social) that build upon each other to establish overall health or changes to that overall health.

Pros

- Improved cardiometabolic health: the indication for shifting dietary intake to include less processed and less refined sugars leads to normalization of metabolic regulatory hormones and increased metabolic flexibility, allowing for lowered levels of oxidative stress and improved overall health
- Weight loss and maintenance: the shift in food portions and proportion of foods coming from refined products, coupled with a lifestyle that encourages greater amounts of physical activity ,the diet can be beneficial in both losing weight and maintaining any weight that has been lost.
- Relatively easy to follow: there is little in terms of inclusion and exclusion that would make the diet restrictive, and given the general popularity of the diet and the ability for it to fit into other dogmatic practices, the diet is very easy

Cons

- Findings from science seem to be an overreach: the reported findings that continually tout benefits seem to ignore other contributing factors to changes in overall health

- Potential for omega-3 and omega-6 imbalance and anti-nutrient interference in metabolism: the higher amounts of nuts and vegetables in the diet can lead to an imbalance in the ratio between omega-3 and omega-6 fatty acids that can cause an inflammatory response, while the presence of anti-nutrients can interfere with digestion of foods and use of nutrients by the body at the cells and tissues of the body. Combined, these might interfere with any benefits arising from following the diet dogmatically

What about other regional or cultural diets that might be followed dogmatically?

When looking into other practices that might influence dietary dogmas, the culture and regional identity of people often serve as a special indicator for food choices and dietary practices. Practices and choices that can be seen both in the secular approach to food, such as with the Mediterranean diet, but also in the form of religious dietary practices found throughout various religions of the world. Whether those practices are vegetarianism, consumption of animal meat butchered in specific ways, or exclusion of specific foods or combination of foods in meals that are being prepared. Dietary approaches can have political and social undertones to their exploitation and utilization in one area of the world, while the same dietary approach might face economic constraints due to prices for obtaining foods in other areas.

It is through these dietary practices that distinct cultures take hold and get expressed through special dietary rules. Specialty diets that vary the strictness of adherence to a diet and/or acceptance of specific foods allow for the development of an us and them attitude. Unfortunately, outside of changes that occur when accepting or transitioning to a "Western" diet, there is limited research into the impact that religious or culturally specific diets have on the health of the individual. Extrapolating from this research, we can stipulate that some of the regionally based and culturally based diets may have a health benefit relative to what we tend to view as a "Western"-style diet. Differences that may be related to the abundance of foods containing metabolic disruptors within foods that comprise the "Western" diet and the impact that these chemicals have on overall health more than the benefit that might come from the regionally-based or culturally-based diets. Even when proponents of following these various diets might advocate for benefits coming from eating vegetarian (see *Go Green*) or that the elimination of intoxicants, stimulants, or alcohol might have on physiological performance and maintaining overall health, to the importance that distinct herbs and spices (see *I need a remedy*), or even following distinct fasting (see *There's a time to eat*) rules can aid in improving body weight and allow one to be healthier in the long run.

Even though there might be issues with strict adherence to regional-based or cultural-based diets, most are not detrimental to health. A claim that can be made and suggested by the simple observation that most diets have been followed for multiple generations, or in some cases, multiple millennia. A fact that may be an indication of metabolic adaptations taking place with n the subpopulations adhering to the dietary practices that allow for benefits to arise more than inherent benefits from the dietary practices themselves.

Nevertheless, some practices may lead to nutritional deficits and inadequacies, especially with strict adherence. Strict observance of the animal slaughtering practices seen in Halal and Kosher practices can increase the risk of iron deficiency or increase the consumption of prepared foods that can lead to excess sodium intake. Those that strictly follow vegan diets (e.g., Seventh Day Adventists, Hindus, or Buddhists) may have deficiencies similar to what is seen in others that follow a vegan dogmatic diet (i.e., vitamin B12, calcium, iron, zinc, selenium, omega-3 fatty acids) along with an imbalance in the ratio of omega-6-to-omega-3 fatty acids).

Take-home message

What can we say about the Mediterranean diet or region-based or culture-based diets? For the Mediterranean diet, there are a host of health and wellness benefits that have been attributed to the Mediterranean diet. However, what

Ancel Keys and other early proponents of the diet and subsequent acolytes seem to forget is that the Mediterranean food and culture are embedded within the history of those living in the region. A dogmatic diet that is incorporated into the wider expression of lifestyles and traditions, religions, and cultural backgrounds and is not simply dietary patterns, lists of ingredients, or cooking recommendations that can be followed decontextualized from the historical background, food quality, and lifestyle habits associated with the people of the region. The true ideals and dogmas of the Mediterranean diet should go beyond the "dietary dogma" of what is included, excluded, or how food is prepared to also take into account the various factors that interact with each other to develop the health and wellness or improvements in overall health that are widely ascribed to the diet without consideration for changes in other lifestyle factors or the interaction that lifestyle and physiological responses have for the improvements noted by others utilizing the dietary dogmatic practice beyond the traditional population living in the Mediterranean area.

While for the other regional and culturally based diets, the reported benefits that are noted appear to align with reported benefits and risks seen with secular diets that are similar. Yet, there is no reason why someone should terminate following such dietary practices, so long as they are able to meet their individual needs for nutrients to ensure proper health and wellness. The use of dietary practices as a means to find belonging, as long as not harmful, offers greater benefits to the individual's psychological well-being relative to the sense of well-being offered through exclusion or rejection from the community. However, at the same time, the community should limit punitive actions for selection to waiver from the strictness of dietary restrictions if the restrictions might cause harm if followed.

For every season, a time to eat...

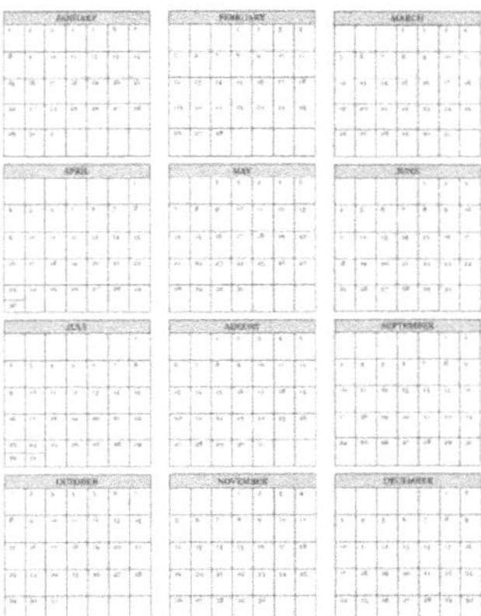

The idea of fasting as a dogmatic dietary practice is as old as religious practices. The entire concept of intermittent fasting, or fasting in general, is not a new concept and has been around for thousands of years. As it has been used as a means to reach a state of greater spiritual awareness. We see this practice of fasting-style diets as an integral part of times of atonement of religions like Judaism and Christianity, as part of times for spiritual renewal and reflection of religions like Islam, Buddhism, Hinduism, and Christianity, as part of interconnectedness with the spiritual worlds of many indigenous religions.

An extension of such fasting has been noted within medical treatment since antiquity, with many Egyptian, Greek, Indian, Persian, and Roman physicians having fasts as being a practice used to heal the body. A practice that comes from observations that during periods of illness, hunger and appetite might be weaker or non-existent, with the conclusion being that the body desires a fast as part of the healing process. The idea of the incorporation of fasting as a potential option for disease was first reported in the earliest peer-reviewed medical journals, and treatment was seen in medicine in the late 1800s. With intermittent fasting being reported on in several books by the turn of the 20th century, becoming a popular dieting trend similar to the fad diets of Banting (low-glycemic/low-carbohydrate diet), Kellogg (vegan whole-grain diet), and Salisbury (low-carbohydrate, high-protein diet) meant to be curative of diabetic conditions (Banting and Salisbury) or digestive conditions (Kellogg and Salisbury) with a side benefit of reducing of fat mass of the individual.

Moving forward to today, the practice of fasting continues, whether for religious observations or as part of a medical treatment. However, fasting-style diets only for aesthetic and body compositional purposes are relatively new and seem to be gaining in popularity. And while we tend to not think of the fasting diets as a proportional diet, there are several aspects of proportional diets that get embedded into the dogmatic practices with these diets quickly becoming one of the more popular ways to establish nutrient and Caloric restrictions in the pursuit of weight loss. Yet, even with a growing body of evidence that supports its use and a long tradition across multiple religions, there are many that simply see these diets as a fad.

To counter this last point, proponents of fasting follow and preach the adage that fasting is easy enough to follow; simply don't eat food for a period of time, and it can easily be incorporated into one's lifestyle and used for prolonged periods. But just as with anything that seems easy, we try to overcomplicate it by attempting to oversimply, as there is not a single means for performing a fasting-style diet. So, let's start by getting some common terms used within this dietary practice. For some proponents of this diet, it means limiting when food is eaten throughout the day; this should be called **time-**

restricted feeding. For others, it means cycling between restricted or nonconsumption of nutrients that is followed by normal consumption, best known as **intermittent fasting**. Similar to intermittent fasting is the idea of **alternate-day fasting,** where one would flip between fasting one day and eating normally the next. And there is even a third way to look at this idea, where dieting takes on the form of prolonged fasts where minimal nutrients are consumed; this is also called **dieting-mimicking fasting**. We traditionally look at this style of dieting as a means to improve metabolic health, not the popular belief that diets are related to weight loss, even though having a focus primarily on weight loss has recently become more prevalent.

Is it intermittent fasting or time-restricted eating?

Intermittent fasting is a weekly breakdown of dieting that alternates a day with limited to no food intake followed by a day of normal food intake; see figure Fasting1. With the most popular being the 5:2 program of 5 days eating and 2 days fasting each week. Interestingly, this type of food restriction follows a similar pattern that many religious fasting observations follow, and these religious observations may serve as the origin of what we consider intermittent fasting to be. Intermittent fasting is a pattern of dieting where you consume no food or very little food that is then followed by days of normal feeding. Regardless of the method (no food or very little food), the idea is to generate a repeatable pattern of fasting and feeding that has severe restrictions followed by normal feeding. The combination of fasting with restriction of nutrients (e.g., low-carbohydrate diet) during feeding has the potential to be an effective means for improving health and causing greater total weight loss than simple Caloric restriction or low-carbohydrate diets.

Figure Fasting1. Examples of how one might establish an intermittent fasting schedule for a week.

Mon	Tues	Wed	Thurs	Fri	Sat	Sun
Fast	Fast	Eat normal	Fast	Fast	Eat normal	Eat normal
Restrict	Restrict	Eat normal	Eat normal	Restrict	Restrict	Eat normal
Fast	Fast	Eat Normal	Restrict	Restrict	Fast	Eat normal

This is different from time-restricted feeding, even if we will commonly flip the terms. Time-restricted feeding is a mechanism of timing when you eat into specific times of the day; see figure Fasting2. The most popular forms for time-restricted feeding are the 12:12, 8:16, and 4:20 programs. In these diet plans, you will eat all of your food for a day, once a day within the shorter time block, followed by a longer time block of fasting. Such as a 4:20 plan using a 4-hour block of time to eat, followed by fasting for the remainder of the day. Or the 8:16 plan, you block off 8 hours for food consumption, typically broken into 2 four-hour blocks, and then will fast for the other 16 hours of the day. While in the 12:12 you block off 12-hours for food consumption into 3 four-hour blocks, usually morning block, mid-day block, and evening block, followed by extended fast overnight. In the eating blocks, you are not technically restricted from eating, but if combined with nutrient restriction, especially following a ketogenic diet, it can be used both for improving health as well as an effective means for weight loss. But it is effective only as long as the fasting block goes uninterrupted. Interestingly, if one were to follow a diet using "three square meals" a day without snacking between meals, they would in fact be following a time-restricted feeding diet.

Of these popular methods, the closest time-restricted feeding to an actual intermittent fasting would be the 4:20 plan, but even then, it is not technically intermittent fasting. This might sound like intermittent fasting, based on how many discuss the topic, but it is not truly intermittent fasting.

Given the understanding of what intermittent fasting and time-restricted feeding happen to be, let's examine what evidence we have as to how it may work.

Figure Fasting2. Examples for how one might be able to break the day (24 hours) into fasting and eating based on time-restricted eating for the day.

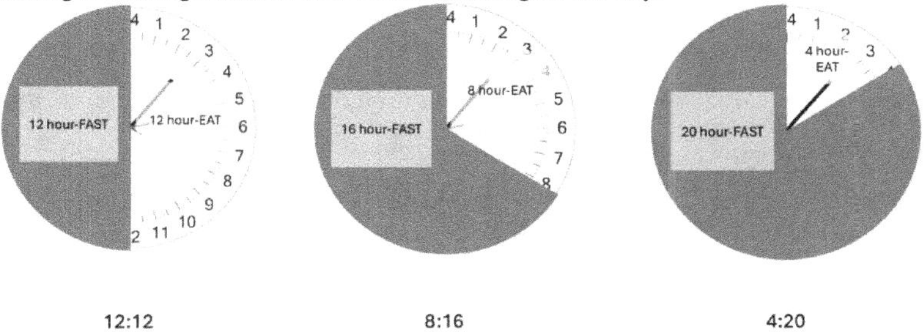

What can we say are the benefits based on scientific evidence?

Before getting into all the benefits, we must acknowledge a caveat in our understanding. The majority of evidence that provides evidence of benefit comes from animal studies, and there is limited evidence about safety or attrition from long-term use of any of the fasting-style diets.

First, it is important to acknowledge that there is no single way to perform intermittent fasting or time-restricted feeding, and thus the summary of how it might work will vary based on methods. Regardless of the methods, the few studies of humans have shown that both intermittent fasting and time-restricted feeding were effective for reducing body mass and fat mass. This is not surprising, yet what is surprising and in agreement with postulates put forth in the book and elsewhere is that loss occurred even when there was no overall restriction in nutrient or Calorie intake on a daily basis. The loss appeared to be differential when the restriction utilized a combination of restrictions, such as when restricting carbohydrates within the intermittent fasting or the time-restricted feeding pattern of feeding. The mechanism that has been proposed for how loss is achieved using intermittent fasting or time-restricted feeding is through an increase of fatty acid oxidation and the generation of ketone bodies for use in generating energy for the body. As the weight loss appears to be comparable to weight loss experienced following other dieting mechanisms that increase fatty-acid oxidation rates (i.e., low-carbohydrate and ketogenic diets).

Along with weight loss, there is a proposed action related to beneficial changes in cardiovascular functions, gastrointestinal functions, and the regulation of glucose levels when following either intermittent fasting or time-restricted feeding. The result of these changes is an improvement in overall health for the volunteers in the studies. In which the cellular and molecular mechanisms by which intermittent fasting improve health and counteract disease processes involve cellular responses that enhance mitochondrial health and repair from reactive oxidative species (ROS) and oxidative stress while also promoting mitochondrial plasticity and mitochondrial-biogenesis (more total mitochondria) and long-lasting positive metabolic effects. A result that leads to improved aerobic functions and normalization of metabolic flexibility for individuals that were following the intermittent fasting or time-restricted feeding diet pattern. All of the cellular responses are matched by improvements in insulin and leptin sensitivity, normalization of adiponectin and other adipokines, and an overall "beigeing" of white adipose tissue during and following the intermittent fasting or time-restricted feeding intervention. When discussing "beigeing" of white adipose, the indication of changing fat metabolism to improve hormonal signals that lead to improved health by reduction of inflammation hormones and increases of anti-inflammatory signals. The effect of the change leads to a continuation of improvements in overall health and takes the person from a condition of fatness and moves them toward a state of fitness; see figure Fasting3.

Figure Fasting3. Changes in physiological state and health status that might occur coming from the use of intermittent fasting (IF) or time-restricted feeding (TRF).

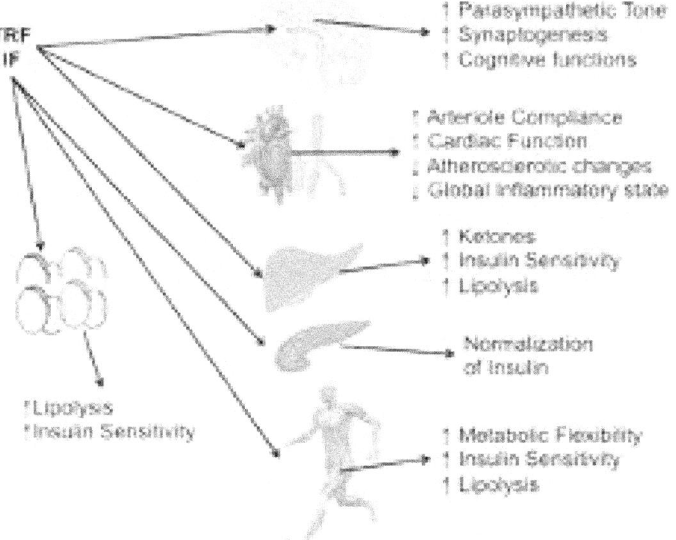

Yet, the mechanisms by which all responses take place have, to date, not been revealed in totality. As such, most of the conclusions reflect back on studies that involve restriction of nutrients (i.e., low-carbohydrate and ketogenic diets, vegetarian) or based on responses seen following the combination of dietary restriction combined with prolonged endurance training. The primary mechanisms appear to be based on carry-over effects from the fasting days to the feeding days. One effect is that the average restriction lead to, on average, a reduced intake of 25-30% below normal Caloric intake. This reduced Caloric intake reflects a nutrient deficiency that leads to alterations in fatty acid oxidation and ketone body generation. This results in a reduction in oxidative stress and formation of ROS (free radicals), normalization of insulin and leptin sensitivity, improved metabolic flexibility at skeletal muscles, and alteration of adipokins, figure Fasting3.

Dieting-Mimicking Fasting

Dieting-Mimicking fasting is a form of dieting that attempts to combine the tenets of Caloric restriction with the tenets of time-restricted feeding and intermittent fasting into one program. This dogmatic approach to dieting is different from intermittent fasting and time-restricted feeding as it allows you to eat small amounts of food throughout the day. The small meals are designed with the intention to provide specific amounts of the carbohydrates, lipids (fats), and proteins necessary for proper metabolism without needing to extract the missing nutrients from the tissues of the body. Although both dieting-mimicking fasting and intermittent fasting have been linked with improvement in metabolic health, the proponents of following this diet appear to indicate that mimicking prolonged fasts can have benefits beyond metabolic health and have pointed to possible extension of life span from following this diet. However, we must be very careful supporting this claim, as it has only been shown in rodents and quality of life was not considered. Additionally, there are several lifestyle factors that come into play when discussing life span for the individual, and dieting is only one of them.

What do we know about the benefits and costs of fasting?

To start addressing this point, it is important to know that benefits and risks are not universal, and men and women show differences in responses based on the style of fasting.

Even with differences, it is important to stipulate similar responses for men and women for the adherence rates to the diet, relative weight loss and/or body compositional changes, to any improvement in cardiovascular functions, and reduction in total cholesterol and LDL. Responses indicate that both men and women can benefit from following a fasting-style diet. However, an interesting point of contention has been noted. When examining the published results from intermittent fasting diet research, women and men tend to respond quite differently to intermittent fasting-style diets. There are differences in responses that are not noticed in the other fasting-style diets, whether that be time-restricted feeding, alternate-day fasting, or dieting-mimicking fasting.

Differences that arise during and after intermittent fasting include dissimilar responses associated with diabetic indices (changes in levels of insulin and glucose) and the amount of fatty acids circulating around the body in our blood. Men who have metabolic issues have a response that makes them appear more "normal," while women tend to have a response that is not a response... meaning women tend to not normalize the signals of diabetes when using a fasting-style diet. Women also show a reduction in metabolic rate, while men can actually show an increase during fasts, while afterward, women show a "linear" return to eating while men show a delay when they return to eating. There is speculation that the differences seen between men and women have been associated with possible differences in how individuals respond to ketogenic metabolism more than dieting itself. Meaning that we should expect to see potential differences in response to any style of diet that involves excessive amounts of restriction, regardless of how we might label that dietary pattern.

This all leads to the obvious question: **why? Why would men and women respond differently to diets that utilize fasting?** Most of us would immediately answer, "It has to be because of Testosterone!" or "No duh, it's because of Estrogen!" The typical culprits that are used to explain the differences we see physiologically between our socially identified genders. While there are differences in these hormones, the responses that we see during periods of intermittent fasting or excessively restrictive dieting go beyond just these two hormones; see Table Fasting1.

Table Fasting1. Hormones known to impact metabolism and overall health status that are changed by fasting.

Hormone	Noted change from fasting and outcome	Hormone	Noted change from fasting and outcome
Adenosine	Increased: fatigue, moodiness, hunger	Adenosine Monophosphate Kinase (AMPk)	Increased: fatigue, hunger
Adiponectin	Increase: hunger, altered glucose metabolism by changes of insulin sensitivity	Adiposin	Decrease: altered fat metabolism and metabolic characteristics of fat cells
Adrenal Androgens (DHEA-S)	Decreased: variable responses associated with fat mass and fat-free mass	Adrenaline (Epinephrine)	Increased: variable responses, altered glucose metabolism and mobilization of fats for fuel
Cortisol	Increased: altered inflammation response, altered glucose metabolism and mobilization of amino acids from proteins for fuel	Dopamine	Increased: moodiness, hunger drive
Estrogen	Variable changes: altered reproductive functions, altered response to tissue growth signal at fat-free mass	Ghrelin	Increased: hunger, altered GH production
Glucagon	Increased: hunger, altered glucose metabolism and mobilization of glucose from glycogen and increased gluconeogenesis at the liver	Glucagon-like Peptide	Decreased: hunger, altered digestive functions, altered glucose metabolism through inability to block glucagon actions

Growth Hormone (GH)	Variable response: increased small GH to mobilize fats for fuel and alter glucose metabolism; decrease large GH to alter growth at fat-free tissues of the body	**Insulin**	Decreased: hunger, altered glucose metabolism, reduced growth signals at fat-free and fat mass
Insulin-like Growth Factor (IGF)	Decreased: reduced growth response at fat-free mass	**Interleukins (IL)**	Variable responses: IL-1, IL-2 reduced with reduced inflammation response; IL-6, IL-10 increased with reduced inflammation leading to normalization of glucose metabolism and improved metabolic flexibility
Irisin	Variable response: altered glucose metabolism by changes in insulin and glucagon sensitivity	**Leptin**	Decreased: hunger, altered glucose metabolism through changes in insulin and glucagon sensitivity, increase fat breakdown and mobilization of fat for fuel
Myokines	Variable response: reduced growth response at fat-free mass, altered glucose metabolism by changes in insulin and glucagon sensitivity	**Noradrenaline (Norepinephrine)**	Increased: variable responses, altered glucose metabolism and mobilization of fats for fuel

Obestatin	Decreased: hunger, altered fat metabolism	Orexin	Increased: hunger, altered hypothalamus and pituitary functions reducing overall hormone responses regulating metabolic rates
Osteocalcin	Increased: hunger, altered bone metabolism	Oxyntomodulin	Reduced: hunger, altered digestive functions
Pancreatic Peptide Tyrosine-Tyrosine	Reduced: hunger, altered digestive function	Resistin	Reduced: improved cardiovascular functions
Retinol Binding Protein-4 (RBP-4)	Increased: altered glucose metabolism through changes in insulin sensitivity	Testosterone	Variable changes: altered reproductive functions, altered growth response at fat-free tissues
Thyroid Hormone (T$_3$ and T$_4$)	Reduced: altered aerobic metabolism, reduced growth response at fat-free tissues	Serotonin	Decreased: moodiness, hunger drive
Visfatin	Variable response: altered fat metabolism, altered fat cell metabolic characteristics		

Of all the hormones that might impact the differences seen, the response to the hormone Leptin seems to have the greatest impact, even when there are changes seen in the sex steroids during periods of fasting. Because Leptin has a greater impact on metabolism in women than men, any change in Leptin will, by extension, have a greater impact on women than men. When following fasting or excessive restriction of nutrients, the responses seen in women (the reduced metabolic rate, the linear return to normal eating) are directly related to what Leptin regulates (hunger, metabolic rate), which helps explain why women show differences in their responses relative to what is seen in men.

There are also noted changes in pituitary and hypothalamic hormones that occur through the duration of the intermittent fasting period, all linked to changes in Leptin and other adipokines (fat-cell-derived hormones). Changes that will directly impact metabolic rate through regulation of the production and release of growth hormone (GH) along with regulatory hormones (e.g., thyroid stimulating hormone (TSH)); see figure Fasting4, can have a negative impact on overall metabolism and metabolic rates. Responses from the pituitary reduce the amounts of the larger versions of the GH molecule and TSH that allow for a reduction in metabolic rate to parallel the reduction in nutrients coming from the fast.

Figure Fasting4. Impact that restriction of nutrition has on hormone concentration, pituitary functions and metabolic rates.

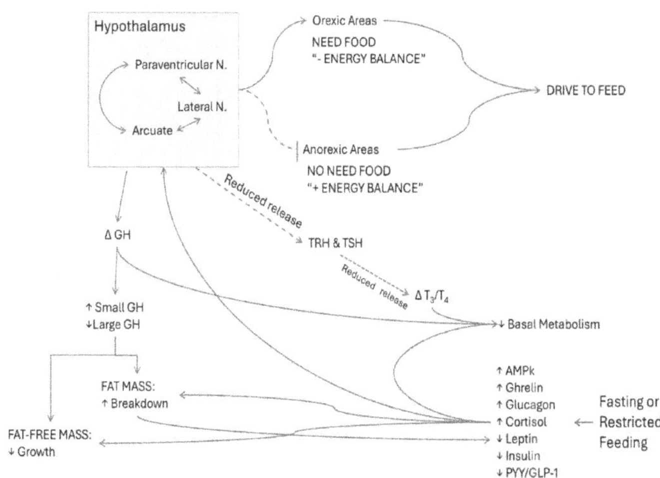

Because women have greater responses to Leptin and adipokines relative to men, the impact that these hormones have on the women's pituitary would lead to a significant impact on the functions of the pituitary. Along with adipokines, the levels of amino acids, glucose, ketones, and fatty acids in circulation also function as key regulators to the type of GH being produced and released by the pituitary. During fasting, changes in adipokines and these metabolites lead to greater amounts of the smaller version of GH being produced and released. A response that is associated with the reduced building of tissues, mood swings, and greater breakdown of fats throughout the body and improving glucose levels by assisting the actions of Glucagon that happen when fasting causes a drop of glucose. Changes in hormone concentrations can be less pronounced in women relative to men, accompanied by differences in responses to these hormone, with women possibly showing a lower degree of response than men.

The changes in hormones coming from the pituitary and hypothalamus will also directly alter the hormones that regulate reproductive functions. Changes in reproductive hormones can lead to men showing an increased level of Testosterone and receptors, along with Luteinizing Hormone (LH), a key regulator of testosterone production. While changes for women can lead to a reduction in ovary functions and Estrogen levels due to lower amounts of Follicle Stimulating Hormone (FSH), there is no change in LH, which is all linked to another regulatory hormone called Kisspeptin. Kisspeptin is a hormone coming from the hypothalamus that controls how much FSH will be produced and released by the pituitary. When Leptin (and other adipokines) drastically change, the hypothalamus slows the amount of Kisspeptin being released, which in turn reduces FSH release. A consequence that impacts women at a much higher rate than men, as the function of Kisspeptin is more pronounced in women than in men, leading to greater changes in the sex hormones in women than in men. Also, when fasting, the circulating metabolites, especially fatty acids, that inhibit testosterone production in males drop, a drop not seen in women that further helps explain some differences occurring.

Expanding the discussion beyond the fasting-style diets, differences we see in response to hormones like Leptin and other adipokines can explain why weight loss in postmenopausal women can be quite difficult. Additionally, the differences in hormonal responses not only explain the differences that occur during fasting but also the differences that occur during normal food intake. Variations that can help us understand the recognized differences that are seen in the general nutritional recommendations for men and women. Along with explaining why the equations we use to estimate metabolic rates have an equation for men and for women.

What can we say about fasting-style diets?

Many popular fad diets (i.e., the HCG diet, the Sleeping Beauty diet, the Cabbage diet) stipulate the positive effects of fasting for weight loss. Weight loss that primarily occurs through the result of extreme nutrient restriction, restrictions that can become dangerous to one's overall health. Yet, proponents of these fasting diets would say that it is not extreme fasting that causes weight loss but other factors, namely changes in metabolic rates that come from the diet, that are the primary cause of weight loss.

But fasting can have benefits, as long as the focus of the fast is not to cause excessive negative restrictions on food that can harm one's overall health or trigger food avoidance issues. There are beneficial metabolic responses to following a fasting-style diet that include moderate weight loss, improved metabolic health, and improved cardiovascular health. However, these benefits do not appear to be universal across all of the styles of fasting diets, especially in regard to weight loss. There are noted differences in the responses that we see from time-restricted eating, alternate-day fasting, or dieting-mimicking fasting compared to the responses seen from intermittent fasting. Differences that appear to be based on the gender (or biological sex) of the person and the influence that this individual characteristic has on our responses to the hormones that regulate metabolism and possibly body weight. For men, using any fasting-style diet can be beneficial for both metabolic health and for weight loss. For women, the use of time-restricted eating and possibly alternate-day fasting has shown greater benefit than the other fasting-style diets.

Pros
- Generally easy to follow with a variety of methods that can be employed to allow for fasting with everyone showing benefits from time-restricted feeding and alternate-day fasting.

- Improvements in metabolic health, including increased insulin and leptin sensitivity.
- Improvements in cardiovascular health, including reduced blood pressures and better heart functions.
- Improvements in body composition and weight management
- If following proportional guidelines during times of eating, there is no risk for deficiencies that might occur in other dietary practices

Cons

- Benefits may not be universal for everyone if using true intermittent fasting versus the other forms of the fasting-style diets, with women having a lower rate of beneficial responses relative to men when following intermittent fasting
- Can become socially restrictive and have poor attrition rate in the long term
- High risks for hypoglycemia during fasting, especially if coupled with exercise during the fasting period
- High risk for developing eating disorder issues if correlating the restrictions in eating with the necessity to establish a Caloric deficit.

Take-home message:

Overall, intermittent fasting and time-restricted feeding appear to be just as efficient as other diet dogmas (i.e., low-carbohydrate and ketogenic diets, vegan) at modifying weight and changes in metabolic health. Additionally, the changes in long-term health are also very similar to other dietary methods with parallelity to metabolic changes seen when diet is combined with exercise. It must be stated, even with these plausible benefits, there are almost no long-term studies or studies with follow-up on continuation of benefit following the termination of the study. Taken together, we must be very careful to accept the purported benefits of intermittent fasting or time-restricted feeding or dieting-mimicking fasting as a panacea for improving health or inducing greater weight loss relative to other dieting methods.

Go green or go home...

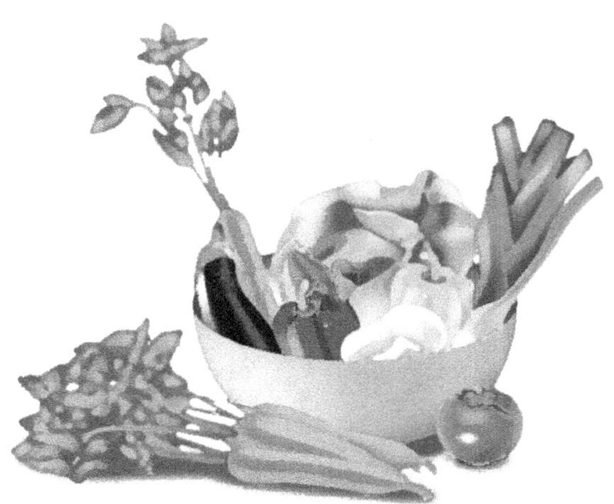

Plant-Based Diets

The idea of using a plant-based diet is not a new phenomenon. There are encyclopedias of dietary advice from antiquity to modern day that follow the recommendation of increasing consumption of vegetables and fruits as a means to alleviate any number of health ailments. The central tenet of the diet is one that can treat everything from heart disease, diabetes, and digestive issues to being the only way to get rid of gout. A philosophy that led to one of the first mass-produced "fad" health foods on record, Kellogg's Corn Flakes. A product that arose from Kellogg's perspective was that the only way to be healthy was to follow a vegan, low-sugar diet with ample amounts of physical activity. A perspective that he translated into his health sanitarium diet of the late 1800s, a diet that we can trace the entire lineage of a staple in the grocery store and the American diet to, one that we take for granted today ... Breakfast Cereals.

Ignoring the past, as we tend to do, we see a growing amount of popularity in a host of plant-based diets over the last half-century. Growth in popularity has been associated with a number of reasons. Some have voiced that plant-based diets are popular and should be followed because of the positive environmental impact that they have versus the other dogmatic diets. In particular, proponents will point to the lower carbon footprint that comes from the plant-based diets. Some argue plant-based diets are popular and should be followed because of a litany of health benefits that supposedly come from the diet. Proponents of this dogmatic dietary practice rely on the evidentiary suggestions that consuming plant-based diets is associated with a reduced risk of many non-communicable diseases (e.g., cardiovascular disease (CVD) and hypertension, metabolic syndrome, neurodegenerative diseases, and cancer). While for others, they get the sense that a plant-based diet is something that links to our evolutionary heritage. A premise based on a false understanding of what humans have been eating over the length of human history or an implication that evolution has stopped and that modern dietary practices are an antithesis to evolutionary pressures. Talking points that lead to a host of apostles touting the benefits of the plant-based diets through a variety of dogmatic practices, with two major sects: vegetarians and vegans.

Before getting into the various aspects of what these diets might do for us, I think it important to get some definitions out of the way first, as it will explain the differences in what is or is not allowed in the diet; See table Green1.

A **vegetarian** is simply a person that's going to eat things that do not contain animal meat. Within this, we have different types of vegetarians based on what they might add to their plant-based diet. We have **lacto-vegetarians,** who will consume animal-derived milk products within their plant-based diet but will not eat any animal meat. There are **ovo-vegetarians,** those that will consume eggs along with their plant-based diet but no other animal meat. A combination of these styles leads to the **lacto-ovo-vegetarians,** those who also consume milk and eggs within their no-animal-meat diets. Finally, there are the **pesco-vegetarians,** who will be vegetarians that will add fish to their d et to obtain additional protein not available from eating solely vegetables. But then we have very strict vegetarians, known as **vegans,** who will not use any products or eat any foods that come from an animal. For a vegan, life is derived from having a plant-based existence, meaning that for dietary practices a vegetarian might allow within their dietary dogma things like honey, whereas a vegan will not.

The central tenet of the plant-based diet is not focusing on how much or how little food is consumed, but which food groups are being emphasized (i.e., fruits, vegetables, grains) and which are being eliminated (i.e., meat, dairy). A tenet that has a lot of proponents instilling that their diet will be healthier for you, regardless of the sect within the dogma that one chooses to follow.

Table Green1. Foods and food sources that would be acceptable based on the different plant-based diets.

Dietary Practice	Acceptable Food Sources	Secondary Food Sources	Can processed foods be present in the diet? (Yes/No)
Vegetarian	Fruits Vegetables Nuts Legumes Cereals (grains) Vegetable oils and butters Nut oils and butters Non-Dairy Beverages Non-Dairy Beverage-derived foods	Honey Nutritional Yeast	YES

Ovo-vegetarian	Fruits Vegetables Nuts Legumes Cereals (grains) Vegetable oils and butters Nut oils and butters Non-Dairy Beverages Non-Dairy Beverage-derived foods	Honey Nutritional Yeast Eggs	YES
Lacto-vegetarian	Fruits Vegetables Nuts Legumes Cereals (grains) Vegetable oils and butters Nut oils and butters Non-Dairy Beverages Non-Dairy Beverage-derived foods	Honey Nutritional Yeast Animal- derived milk Animal-derived butter and dairy foods	YES
Lacto-Ovo-vegetarian	Fruits Vegetables Nuts Legumes Cereals (grains) Vegetable oils and butters Nut oils and butters	Honey Nutritional Yeast Eggs Animal- derived milk Animal-derived butter and dairy foods	YES
Pesco-vegetarian	Fruits Vegetables Nuts Legumes Cereals (grains) Vegetable oils and butters Nut oils and butters Non-Dairy Beverages Non-Dairy Beverage-derived foods	Honey Nutritional Yeast Fish, Shell-fish	YES

Vegan	Fruits Vegetables Nuts Legumes Cereals (grains) Vegetable oils and butters Nut oils and butters Non-Dairy Beverages Non-Dairy Beverage-derived foods	Nutritional Yeast	YES

Yet, because of how the dogma and tenets are formed, the plant-based diets succumb to a number of myths and misconceptions that other dogmatic practices do not. The tenets insist that a plant-based diet is inherently healthier because of the focus on plants but at the same time has limited focus on how the food is prepared, cooked, or if processed foods are being excluded. Factors that we know have an impact on exposing the person to metabolic disruptors and can impact health or benefits that are touted as coming from plant-based diets. Benefits that due to oversimplification and excessive exposure to messaging tend to become a means of avoidance of this dogmatic diet by people that choose a different dogmatic diet. But then there are a host of misconceptions that can come into play, especially for people that wish to follow this dietary practice but are excessively active or athletic. Topics that were part of a prolonged conversation that I had with a former student in August of 2023 that led to three key points to remember about forming your plant-based dietary practice:

1. There is no reason to not use a plant-based diet if that is what you would select to use, but we need to understand the social exclusion that can develop from following ever-restrictive plant-based diets. It can become difficult to have social gatherings outside the home when friends and family are not following plant-based dietary dogmas. This can also lead to restaurants that offer plant-based options that are simply the removal of the meat from a meal that does not offer the same quality meal as what can be obtained from a complete plant-based meal.

2. Make sure that you are combining protein sources to get complete proteins so that you meet your needs for essential amino acids (especially methionine), along with getting enough creatine, taurine, or carnitine to offset what is being used each day. Creatine can be a problem as we need 6 grams per day and it can be difficult to obtain in our diet without animal meat, especially white meat.

3. Look for various sources of foods (unprocessed, processed, powders) to meet nutrient balance, but limit total amounts of processed foods to limit exposure to metabolic disruptors. Plant-based dieters that are excessively restrictive can quickly become malnourished; a lot of the weight loss that comes from plant-based diet severely restricting the amount and variety of nutrients being consumed, thus weight loss may not be beneficial but is symptoms of malnourishment.

What does science say about the benefits of following a plant-based diets?

What do we know about vegetarian and vegan diets as they relate to the ability to control metabolic health related to weight loss? Questions that are being addressed because most of the people are going to be following dietary dogmas either to regulate body weight or regulate metabolic health.

There are some correlations that indicate following a plant-based diet will lead to changes in neuronal health by increasing insulin sensitivity, reducing reactive oxidative species (ROS), and neuroinflammation. Changes in neuron functions lead to greater neuroplasticity and growth signals that reduce the risks for neurodegenerative disease (i.e., dementia, Alzheimer's disease, Parkinson's disease) and have the potential to improve both learning and motor functions. There is some evidence through correlations to indicate there's an increase in metabolic flexibility, an increase in insulin sensitivity, and a change in myokine signaling within the skeletal muscle. Changes that lead to improved metabolic health and reduced risk for developing metabolic syndrome or treating health issues associated with metabolic syndrome. There are noted improvements in cardiovascular functions that are associated with correlations that indicate there is a reduction in inflammation through the control of the hormone C-reactive protein, a hormone that triggers hypertension (high blood pressure), along with a reduction of LDL and triglyceride levels. The combination leads to a reduced atherosclerosis (hardening of the arteries) that allows for reduced blood pressure and, by association, improved heart functions.

Metabolically, following a plant-based diet has been associated with improved pancreas functions. Improvements that are reflected in the normalization of Insulin and Glucagon signaling in response to fluctuations in glucose levels in the body. This is accompanied by increased Insulin, Leptin, and GLP-1 sensitivity, along with improved glucose metabolism and reduction of glycosylated hemoglobin, leading to resolving symptoms of metabolic syndrome (i.e., diabetic issues). There is also an increase in breaking down fats to be used as fuel for the body. The change in fat metabolism leads to a decrease in building fats within adipose tissue and a reduction in fat mass. A combination of changes that leads to an improved Leptin sensitivity along with an alteration in adipokine signaling that changes the activation of macrophages and the reduction in inflammation and improved immune function throughout the body.

At the liver, there tends to be an increase in Insulin sensitivity, a reduction in non-alcoholic fatty acid liver syndromes, improved response to GLP-1 and Glucagon that better regulates gluconeogenesis and assists with normalizing blood glucose levels associated with metabolic health. Additionally, there tends to be a change in liver metabolism leading to improved clearance of lipoproteins (LDL) and with hormonal signaling coming away from the liver that leads to improved metabolic health through increased insulin sensitivity and glucose metabolism that is very similar to the same changes that we see in hormonal signaling coming away from the other insulin-dependent tissues (i.e., adipose tissue and skeletal muscle).

Along with hormonal modifications, there is some evidence that indicates plant-based diets increase the health and function of the gut microbiome. The greater intake of dietary fiber and the fermentable substrates formed by the proliferation of Bacteroidetes include the production of very important short-chain fatty acids, e.g., acetate, propionate, and butyrate. Metabolites from the microbiome that have been shown to reduce blood pressure and have a beneficial impact on modulating inflammation and immune activation. Moreover, long-term use of plant-based diets has also been associated with greater biodiversity microbiota in contrast to the microbiota found in those that eat a less plant-rich diet. With a microbiome in the latter group having poor microbiota-accessible carbohydrates that lead to adverse environmental conditions for the intestinal microbiome that alter other metabolite production, potentially impair our immune function, and increase the risk of developing a chronic inflammation and metabolic diseases.

What about body weight and body composition? As with any of the dogmatic dietary practices, the focus has shifted from one of health benefit to one for aesthetic benefit. In this case, a plant-based diet has the potential for assisting in weight loss and changing body composition (i.e., breaking down fat mass). There are a host of reasons for this benefit; most are due to a deficiency in macronutrient intake coupled with metabolic changes and subsequently changes in hormones that lead to reductions of body mass and fat mass. There is also a potential change in the regulation of hunger based on the increased amount of fiber in the diet leading to a prolonged sense of feeling full and a slowing in the rate of absorption of nutrients from the intestines.

It seems like there's a lot of benefits that come away from following a plant-based diet, but does that automatically mean a healthier diet? This is where we have to focus on most of the benefits associated with the diet coming from correlations more than causal effects. With most of the long-term studies showing benefits being rodent studies and not from humans, where findings in rodents may not transfer directly to humans. And it needs to be said that even though the anecdotes we see in the media might speak of benefits and benefits and benefits without any adverse effects, there are almost as many studies that indicate following a vegetarian or a vegan diet may have adverse effects as there are that show only benefits. Ideas that lead to the question…

What are some of the risks and costs of following a plant-based diet?

First, there is a risk for developing health issues based on the impact of either nutrient deficiencies or excessive exposure to anti-nutrients in the diet. Where the evidence indicates when there is greater restrictiveness in the plant-based diets, especially within veganism, there is an exponentially higher risk of hemorrhagic stroke and spontaneous bone fractures. There is also the potential impact the excessively restricted plant-based diets have on breastfeeding women and on the growth and maturation in children that come from a range of vitamin and mineral deficiencies.

These nutrient deficiencies, see Table Green2, are primarily going to be from nutrients that are normally obtained from animal meats or derived products that we consume in our diet, or from supplements that would come from animal products. The most common deficiencies are with vitamins (i.e., vitamin B_{12}, and vitamin D), along with a host of cations (positive ions). We will also lose out on omega-3 fatty acids, eicosapentaenoic acid (EPA), and docosahexaenoic acid (DHA), and with an overt focus on nuts and other omega-6-rich foods there is an increased risk for a disruption in the 6:1 ratio cap for omega-6 to omega-3 fatty acids. A disruption that has been linked with triggering metabolic inflammation.

Table Green2. Summary of potential nutrient deficiencies that can come about due to plant-based diets.

Macromolecule Deficiencies	Mineral Deficiencies	Vitamin Deficiencies
Protein	Calcium	Vitamin A
Essential Amino Acids	Iodine	Vitamin B_{12}
(especially Methionine)	Iron	Vitamin D
Taurine	Magnesium	Vitamin E
Creatine	Phosphorus	
EPA	Sodium	
DHA	Zinc	

Then there is the increased chance for deficiencies in essential amino acids, along with the amino acids taurine (necessary for neuron function) and creatine (necessary for cells to do work). Amino acids that we tend to get in high concentrations from animal products or consumption of supplements, which may be missed based on the strictness of the vegetarian diet that we're trying to follow. Protein and amino acid deficiencies can be countered one of two ways. It can be countered by overconsuming pairs of plant materials known to have larger amounts of essential amino acids that, when they are combined together, generate enough "complete proteins" in the diet. If you chose not to overconsume food, then it will require that you utilize supplemental sources of the amino acids and proteins that are lacking in the diet, if the tenets being held to the specific dogma will allow supplementation to be used. The problem with the supplements is that most are going to involve some animal-derived process in generating the supplement that may not be allowed for the vegan that chooses to follow an excessively restrictive diet holding true to every tenet of the vegan dogma.

The reduction in protein intake and deficiencies in amino acids leads to the next risk for those following the plant-based diets. While proponents will stipulate that the weight loss is from fat mass, weight loss will come from all types of body mass, both fat mass and fat-free mass. The degree of loss of fat-free mass is related to the reduced total amount of protein and amino acids contained within the proteins from the diet. The loss of proteins and essential amino acids, along with essential fatty acids and vitamins that are ingested with foods richer in protein, will lead to the loss of nutrients and metabolites necessary for hormone signals required to maintain fat-free mass during periods of weight loss.

Additionally, the excessive consumption of plants can lead to the exposure of substances referenced as **anti-nutrients**, table Green3. While many of the anti-nutrient compounds have the potential for antioxidant effects that can improve overall health, anti-nutrients (e.g., lectin, oxalates, phytic acid or phytates, phytosterols, tannins, saponins, and goitrogens and glucosinolates) can impact absorption of micronutrients in the intestines or alter the bioavailability of vitamins and minerals that can impact our overall metabolism, or in the case of phytosterols, act as an endocrine disruptor.

To cover this point in a little more detail, let's take a step back and define another term, **bioavailability**. While we tend to have a general idea that if I have something in my diet, it will automatically be used by the body, not everything is automatically ready to be used by the body. This is where bioavailability comes into play, as it is the reference given to whether a substance being digested and absorbed is ready to be used by the cells and tissues of the body. And from this idea of bioavailability, we can better understand the deficiency status for someone, even when eating foods known to have high concentrations of that specific nutrient. Which is where anti-nutrients can impact nutrient deficiencies by either changing how much of a nutrient can be digested and absorbed or whether the absorbed nutrient can be biologically available for the cells of our body. To counter the impact that anti-nutrients have, there are a couple of options for those following a plant-based diet. One can either soak or allow seeds and grains to sprout, or boil and cook plant-based foods prior to eating. These actions work to lower the amount of anti-nutrients contained in the foods or lessen the potential impact that anti-nutrients have on the digestion of food and absorption of nutrients within the intestines.

While there are noted metabolic benefits that can arise from a plant-based diet, there are also known metabolic impacts that can have adverse effects on health. First, plant-based diets can lead to exposure to high amounts of estrogen-like endocrine disruptors in the form of phytosterols. Phytosterols are recognized to impact estrogen metabolism in breast tissue, in bones, and potentially interfere with testosterone metabolism. Exposure that leads to an increased risk for estrogen-derived cancers, osteoporotic changes in bone, and potentially a reduced growth response in large fibers in skeletal muscle following resistance training.

Table Green3. Summary of primary anti-nutrients found in higher concentrations in plant-based diets based on food source and potential adverse impact on digestive or metabolic functions of the body.

Anti-nutrient	Food Source	Potential adverse impact
Glucosinolates and Goitrogens	Kale, Brussels Sprouts, Cabbage, Turnip-greens, Chinese Cabbage, Broccoli, Millet, Cassava	Hypothyroidism Inhibit iodine uptake
Lectins	Legumes, Cereal and Grains, Seeds, Nuts, Fruits, Vegetables	Altered gut function Promote inflammation
Oxalates	Spinach, Swiss Chard, Sorrel, Beet-greens, Beet Root, Rhubarb, Nuts, Legumes, Cereals and Grains, Sweet Potatoes, Potatoes	Inhibit calcium absorption Increase kidney stone formation
Phytic Acid or Phytate	Legumes, Cereals and Grains, Amaranth, Quinoa, Millet, Nuts, Seeds	Inhibit absorption of iron, zinc and calcium Antioxidant effect Antineoplastic effects
Phytoestrogens	Soy and soy products, Flaxseeds, Nuts, Fruits, Vegetables	Endocrine disruption Increased risk of estrogen-sensitive cancers
Tannins	Tea, Cocoa, Grapes, Berries, Apples, Stone Fruits, Nuts, Beans, Whole Grains	Inhibit iron absorption Reduction of iron stores

There are several metabolic impacts that have led many to label plant-based diets as being a "good" diet due to the exclusion of various food sources noted to have an adverse impact on overall health, notably consuming processed and ultra-processed foods. As plant-based diets are reported to limit the impact that metabolic disruptors in processed foods might have on our physiology. In which metabolic disruptors have the potential to alter our food drive and reward responses, leading to overconsumption of food, triggering a pro-inflammatory response that can negatively impact sensitivity to Leptin and Insulin leading to poor metabolic health through stimulating growth response in fat tissues combined with reducing growth responses in the musculoskeletal tissues. Yet, as was noted in the table of food sources, all plant-based diets have the potential to include processed foods. A potential for inclusion that has risen with the growing popularity of the plant-based diets and the commercialism that these diets have across the globe. Changes in signaling that mimic the issues that we typically look at originating from metabolic syndrome and overfatness that we are attempting to correct through the use of the plant-based diet. A reminder that just because we might be following a vegan or vegetarian diet does not mean that we're not also having the possibility of consuming metabolic or endocrine disruptors within the plant-based materials.

Along with nutrient issues and impacts on metabolism, there are other risks that followers of the plant-based diets need to worry about. Based on the perception of restrictions in the diet, combined with the self-selection toward plant-based diets there can be a disruption in the psychological drive we have toward food based on the desire to eat or eat specific things that are liked and enjoyed. This is not necessarily the cognitive desires attributed to the bliss point or the reward center response linked to eating; instead, this is the cognitive drive of wanting to eat. There is also the feeling of exclusion due to following the specifics of the plant-based diet. Exclusions that can be excessively burdensome to the point of having the dietary practice feel like punishment when following the more restrictive dogmas within the dietary practices, e.g., the closer to veganism, and that is furthest from a self-selected pattern, the more disruption will occur. This is where the consistent messaging of "good" versus "bad" food choices is not intrinsically selected for, leading to a desire to select the food that we are being forced to avoid, the "bad," over the foods we are being forced to eat, the "good," food.

What can we say about plant-based diets?

Plant-based diets can have benefits, as long as the focus of the diet is not to cause or trigger food avoidance issues. There are beneficial responses, including a reduced risk of developing noncommunicable diseases and possibly weight loss. Yet, these benefits come at a potential cost that includes nutrient deficiency that can disrupt normal metabolic function, the need to overconsume food to ensure appropriate macronutrient load that can cause food aversion issues later on, excessive exposure to plant-derived hormones that act as endocrine disruptors, and potential impact of anti-nutrients on digestive functions.

Pros

- Improved metabolic health: better Insulin and Leptin sensitivity, improved liver metabolism and clearance of lipoproteins and triglycerides, altered glucose metabolism, and improvements in diabetic indices (if the person is a diabetic).
- Improved cardiovascular health: reduced LDL and cholesterol levels have been associated with reduced atherosclerosis and improved blood pressure. Improvements that are associated with improvement in overall heart function.
- Potential for reduced risk for cancer: Plant-based diets offer high amounts of phytochemicals and antioxidants that reduce the relative risk for cancer developments associated with oxidative stress cellular damage.
- Weight loss: not unique to plant-based diets, with deficiencies in macronutrients, there can be weight loss and body compositional changes when following the diet

Cons

- Restrictive: dietary choices can be excessively onerous and can quickly lead to feelings of coercion to continue.
- Socially isolating: the need to plan and structure meals can limit eating outside of the home or outside of vegan and vegetarian restaurants. Myths and misconceptions about plant-based meals can lead to exclusion from group outings or unwillingness to join in meals
- Exposure to metabolic and endocrine: consuming anti-nutrients or phytochemicals in fruits, vegetables, or nuts, and consuming processed mass-produced plant-based foods increases risk for metabolic disruption and health issues associated with inflammation or disruption of estrogen-pathway regulations
- Nutrient Deficiencies and anti-nutrients: the excess intake of anti-nutrient compounds from plants can interfere with absorption of nutrients and may impact metabolic processes. High omega-6 and low omega-3 uptake can lead to chronic inflammation responses. Poor protein and amino acid balance can lead to wasting issues and poor retention of fat-free mass, ion deficit anemia, hypothyroidism, or osteoporotic bone issues

Raw Food Diet

Another form of the plant-based diet that has recently seen a growing level of popularity, at least among the social media feeds of self-proclaimed experts, is the raw food diet. Like the plant-based diet and fasting diets, there are reports from antiquity about physicians advising patients to eat higher amounts of raw fruits and vegetables as part of curative treatment for a variety of ailments. The modern ideas of using a raw food diet within medical care can be traced back to the mid-1850s, with anecdotal reports of following a raw fruit diet leading to the "curing of gout," and became more marketed in the early 1900s, with a variety of physicians publishing books that encouraged a diet predominantly of raw fruits and vegetables as a way to cure digestive issues. To this list, the self-proclaimed experts of today have added the aesthetic ideas about health with raw food diets, just like the plant-based diets, being effective for losing weight. In particular, losing fat from a raw food diet. Regardless of the approach for using the raw food, the general premise and central tenet is to form one's diet around eating uncooked foods that predominantly align with the tenets of the plant-based diet, but without the typical restrictions about animal meat or animal-derived foods.

The general principle followed by proponents of the raw food diet is that you will only eat foods, see table Green4, in their raw form. That means foods are not processed, not refined, and if heated or cooked it will always be done below a temperature around 118°F. The rationale provided for this general principle is that cooking and processing foods are antithesis to our evolutionary biology based on observations of the diets of other great apes (e.g., bonobos, chimpanzees, gorillas) that are close evolutionary relatives to humans. A premise that adds an idea that cooking or processing food leads to loss of nutrients (e.g., vitamins, minerals) or that cooking will adversely alter naturally occurring enzymes found in plants that reduce the quality of digestion of the materials being consumed. Outside of losses, the other rationale offered by proponents of this dietary dogma is that heating foods beyond 118°F leads to the generation of compounds with negative effects on the perception of the food (i.e., flavor, texture, or color) or produces toxic compounds. The idea of heating and processing foods generating toxic compounds comes from the formation of hydrocarbons during the Maillard reactions or that cooking acrylamide (e.g., fatty-acid esters, glycidol, acrolein) having been indicated to alter gut microbiota and potentially increase the risk for metabolic diseases and cancers.

Table Green4. Summary of foods that are allowed for a raw food diet.

Allowed Food Sources	Possible Food Sources	Forbidden Food Sources
Raw fruits, vegetables, seeds, nuts Raw animal meat Dried fruits, vegetables Dried and salt-cured meat Freshly made juices Sprouted beans, legumes, and grains Raw and unpasteurized non-dairy beverages Raw and unpasteurized animal-derived dairy Cold-pressed oils Nutritional yeast Seaweeds "Green" food powders Fermented leafy foods	Fermented Beverages Fermented legume-based foods Sun-cured fruits Sun-cured nuts Sun-cured dried meats Plant-derived butters Nut butters	Cooked foods Processed foods Pasteurized animal-derived dairy Pasteurized non-dairy beverages Refined oils Refined sugars Refined flour Coffee Tea Alcohol

What does science say about the benefits to following a raw food diet?

To start, there are reports of positive benefits in cardiovascular health with noted reversal of hypertension for those that had high blood pressure when starting a raw food diet. The primary rationale given for the reversal and for the positive reports on cardiovascular health are similar to what is reported from the plant-based diets. Which includes reduced levels of C-reactive protein, improvements in LDL:HDL ratios by reducing levels of LDL, total cholesterol, and improved triglyceride levels in circulation. Improvements that are associated with normalization and reduction of blood pressures that correlate with improved overall heart function.

Once again, we see similar changes in metabolic health to what is seen from the other plant-based diets. There is a normalization of glucose levels, increased sensitivity to Insulin and Leptin, changes in fat metabolism that lead to an increased use of fats as fuels or within other metabolic processes, a reduction in reactive oxidative species (ROS) and ROS-associated cellular damage, and a reduced risk for non-alcoholic fatty-acid syndrome in the liver. Improved metabolic health and reduced ROS damage that neurologically is associated with reducing or slowing neurodegenerative diseases and improving neuron functions allowing for increased interactions between neurons and growth of the neurons occurring from normal activity in the brain. What is interesting is that even though there are changes in metabolic health, there is minimal evidence to show changes in pancreatic functions related to glucose metabolism.

As with a lot of the dogmatic diets, especially those that become excessively restrictive in nutrients, there is weight loss for those that use a raw food diet as an intervention to cause weight loss. Most of the weight loss that is seen parallels the weight loss seen with plant-based diets, where loss is associated with an increased risk for malnutrition and the need to extract necessary nutrients from tissues and cells of the body where they are stored.

What are the risks and costs of following the raw food diet?

We see parallels to the plant-based diets as they relate to adverse effects and costs of following a raw food diet. It is true that cooking can have an impact on developing some toxic hydrocarbons, cooking foods has been shown to increase the rate of digestion and the amount of nutrient absorption that can occur following digestion. Meaning that the premise that raw food proponents use for a rationale that uncooked foods are easier to digest is not supported and can lead to the greatest downside from following a raw food diet, malnourishment; see Table Green5. While many will look at this malnourishment in regard to the misguided notion of Caloric balance and consuming foods of low Calories, the issue is the imbalance within the nutrient balance that will exist from a raw food diet. Malnourishment comes not only as a side effect of not cooking food but also from eating excessively restricted food sources. The restriction of food can lead to lower ingestion of essential amino acids and possibly omega-3 fatty acids. Along with a lower than required amount of amino acids (i.e., creatine and taurine) necessary for cellular metabolism or an imbalance in the ratio between omega-6 to omega-3 fatty acids in favor of omega-6 that can cause cellular inflammation and poorer immune response.

Table Green5. Summary of potential nutrient deficiencies that can come about due to plant-based diets.

Macromolecule Deficiencies	Mineral Deficiencies	Vitamin Deficiencies
Protein	Calcium	Vitamin A
Essential Amino Acids	Iodine	Vitamin B_3
(especially Methionine)	Iron	Vitamin B_5
Taurine	Magnesium	Vitamin B_7
Creatine	Phosphorus	Vitamin B_{12}
EPA	Sodium	Vitamin D
DHA	Zinc	Vitamin E
		Vitamin K

Additionally, there are deficiencies in micronutrients that are of concern when following a raw food diet. Deficiencies that can arise from either not consuming enough of the nutrient or exposure to a higher-than-normal level of anti-nutrients due to overconsuming vegetables and nuts. Most notably are changes in the absorption and use of cations (positive-charged ions), such as sodium, that are needed for normal cell activity and to keep the body properly hydrated. Changes that impact functions of cells such as heart muscle, neurons, skeletal muscle and even bones. Along with loss of cations associated with cell functions, there is a potential for lower-than-normal amounts of iron being absorbed, leading to poor iron stores and anemia. Lastly, there can be vitamin deficiencies, especially B vitamins (e.g., Niacin (Vit B_3), Pantothenic Acid (Vit B_5), Biotin (Vit B_7), Cobalamin (Vit B_{12})) that have a negative impact on the ability of the cell to regulate energy levels, build both fats and proteins (including several hormones and hemoglobin in red blood cells) and regulate cell life cycles. These vitamin deficiencies that are associated with altered immune functions, fatigue, anemia, and poor maintenance of fat-free mass. The degree of malnourishment is going to be directly related to the severity of restrictions, with news reports from 2023 of a social media influencer dying from malnourishment while following a fruit-only raw food vegan diet. While this report is an extreme case of the negative effects stemming from a raw food diet, the less severe negative effects due to malnutrition include dysregulation of reproductive functions, greater risk in women relative to men that may be associated with the impact of diet on Kisspeptin production and the negative impact that has on regulatory hormones, Follicle Stimulating Hormone and Luteinizing Hormone.

There is one additional concern that those who follow the raw food diet must be concerned about is that plant-based dieters don't... food poisoning and infection. Consuming of raw and unpasteurized animal-derived dairy products increases the chance for exposure to bacterial infections from *E. coli*, *Salmonella*, and *Listeria*.

What can we say about the raw food diets?

Let's start with dispelling one of the primary misconceptions and myths that serve as a basis for following the diet; it is closer to our evolutionary heritage. The primary reason for making the statement comes from selective evidence of observational studies of closest living relatives (e.g., gorillas, chimpanzees, bonobos), where observers indicate higher consumption of fruit and vegetable relative to meat consumption. But an observation and poorly deduced hypothesis ignores the 200,000-plus years of human evolution following the initiation of cooking or the even longer time since the evolutionary split occurred between humans and other great apes. Cooking food does two things. First, there is greater availability of nutrients in foods that can occur from cooking by allowing for greater rates of digestion and absorption and exposure to nutrients that can only come from food sources that must be cooked for safety reasons. The latter goes with the second effect that cooking foods allows for safer foods to consumed through the elimination of toxins and pathogens from foods.

Yet, like most plant-based diets, a raw food diet will provide someone with high quantities of fruits and vegetables that can lead to prolonged senses of feeling full due to high amounts of fiber and limit the exposure to hydrocarbons and sulfates that are generated during the cooking process of animal meats linked with metabolic dysregulation in the intestines and cancers.

Pros

- Improved metabolic health: reduced sugar content can allow for improved Insulin and Leptin sensitivity, improved liver metabolism, and clearance of lipoproteins and triglycerides.
- Improved cardiovascular health: reduced animal-derived fats and trans fats leads to lower amounts of ROS damage and atherosclerosis that can improve blood pressure and overall heart function.
- Weight loss: similar weight loss to other diets that have nutrient imbalances within the diets.

Cons

- Restrictive and socially isolating: dietary choices can be excessively onerous and can quickly lead to feelings of coercion to continue, especially given the need to plan and structure meals.
- Metabolic and endocrine disruption: excess amounts of phytochemicals and plant-based butters can lead to metabolic disruption from phytosterols and processed foods, leading to health issues associated with inflammation or estrogen-pathway regulations.
- Nutrient deficiencies and excessive anti-nutrients: excess anti-nutrient compounds from plants can interfere with absorption of nutrients and may impact metabolic processes, high omega-6 and low omega-3 uptake can lead to chronic inflammation responses, poor protein and amino acid balance can lead to wasting issues and poor retention of fat-free mass, ion deficits can lead to issues of anemia, hypothyroidism, or osteoporotic bone issues.

Take-home message

There are a number of reasons that one might choose a plant-based dietary practice. For some it is not due to health concepts but out of ethical considerations for the treatment of animals; for some it is an ecological choice as they see plant-based diets as being more environmentally friendly. On the health side, plant-based diets have been associated with reduced risk for cardiovascular disease, metabolic syndrome (diabetes), and cancers, along with a potential increase in longevity. Yet, there are potential downsides to using a plant-based diet, coming from nutrient deficiencies; in particular amino acids, vitamin B12, iron, calcium, iodine. There have been recent reports of excessive malnourishment when a plant-based diet becomes restrictive to one type of plant or plant-based product. After deficiencies, there are issues with metabolic and endocrine disruption occurring due to excessive consumption of plant hormones and compounds that can interfere with our metabolism. Even with these limitations, if you can balance food intake and supplement to ensure replacing nutrients that are missed due to focusing on plant-based foods, there is no reason why a plant-based diet cannot be a viable diet.

What about the raw-food diets? Foods consumed following a raw food diet contain a high concentration of vitamins, minerals, and beneficial phytochemicals. Yet, there is limited evidence for greater amounts of bioavailable substances in circulation relative to other diets, due to the negative impact that high exposure to anti-nutrients seems to have on nutrient bioavailability. The raw food diet may not be able to provide sufficient essential amino acids, essential fatty acids (e.g, DHA and EPA), B vitamins, and fat-soluble vitamins (e.g., vitamin A, vitamin D, and vitamin K). Thus, given the higher amounts of adverse effects of raw foods (e.g., anti-nutrients and toxic substances in uncooked food), along with other risk factors associated with excessive malnutrition when compared with other plant-based diets, it would be more suggestible to use a plant-based diet and not the raw food diet.

Have a drink...

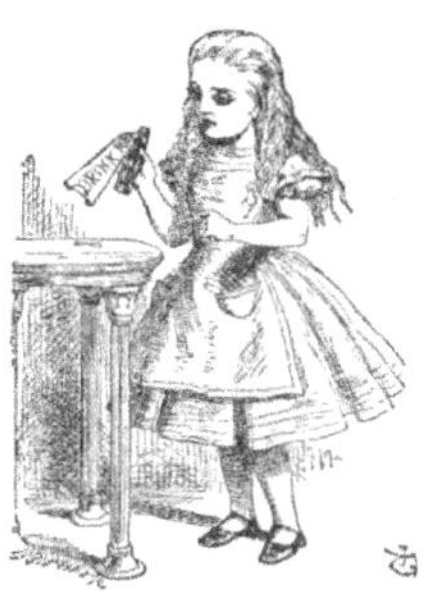

While we tend to think of diets and dogmatic diets as what we eat or don't eat, there is another line of dogmatic practice that takes diets to another realm altogether; **liquid diets**. The foundation of liquid diets, like many of the other dietary practices that have taken over the health and fitness world, comes to us from the medical field. In which liquid diets are regularly used for individuals that cannot physically eat or are preparing for or recovering from surgical procedures. In these instances, a healthcare provider will recommend consuming all nutrients that would normally be found in your food through a liquid. These liquids can be specifically designed to provide the person with the appropriate approach to achieve the nutrient balance necessary and are typically advised for short periods of time.

Yet, there is a growing movement to incorporate a liquid diet beyond these circumstances and for longer than the short period of time that a hea thcare provider might recommend. Anyone that goes to the gym or fitness centers sees the smoothie bars or overhears the bodybuilders and gym rats all tout ng the whey isolate and hydrolyzed protein shakes that you need to drink after your workouts, or the need for the trendiest "antioxidant" berry smoothie to assist in your recovery. You may see these in your social media feeds from companies like Huel or Ka'Chava or AG1, or the social media trends like "WaterTok" or "Oatzempic Challenge" that have been popular, or the continued push to juice or follow a juicing diet that became popular in the 1970s. The general premise that followers of the liquid diets offer is that using the liquid diet will allow you to "cleanse" your body, to detoxify your body; or allow you to reach the body weight and body image that you aim to achieve in a very short period of time.

In case this is all new to you, here are the primary sects of the dogmatic practice:

- Clear liquid diet: most restrictive, and requires all drink to be clear fluids
- Full liquid diet: least restrictive, only requires that what you consume is in liquid form. This can include liquifying and pureeing many animal-derived foods or plant-based diet foods that are generally eaten as solid foods
- Meal replacement liquid diet: similar to a full liquid diet, usually seen with a regimen aligned with changing body weight or body composition. This is the form of the liquid diets that would consume the weight loss protein drinks or the mass-builder protein shakes.
- Detox liquid diet: usually seen as the "juice cleanse" or the "water only" diet that flows from the faulty premise that by changing materials in the intestines there is going to be a cleansing effect on the rest of the body.

The other liquid diet that falls outside the realm of the diets typically thought of as the liquid diets is the alkaline waters. The idea that proponents give for following the alkaline water is that since our body is normally alkaline, the pH of the body ranges from 7.35 to 7.45, we need limit the acid beverages and foods that are consumed, but also consume specialized water that has a pH typically around 9 or consume foods and blended beverages comprised mainly of alkaline foods; see Table Drink1.

Table Drink1. Summary of foods and beverages associated with the alkaline water and diet.

Drinks	Foods	
Electrolyzed Water	Fruits:	Nuts:
Mineral Water	Apples, Apricots,	Chestnuts, Pine nuts
Natural Seltzers	Avocados,	Seeds: Pumpkin
Alkaline Water	Cantaloupe,	Grains:
Herbal Teas	Cherries	Quinoa
Plant-based beverages	Vegetables:	Beans and Legumes:
(Almond milk, Soy	Asparagus, Beets,	Kidney Beans, Red Beans,
milk)	Broccoli, Cabbage,	Soybean and Tofu
Animal-derived	Carrots, Garlic	products
Buttermilk Animal-		
derived Yogurt		

Proponents of the alkaline water and alkaline liquid diet stipulate that using the diet leads toa variety of health benefits: anti-aging, "detoxifying" and digestive "cleansing" properties, immune boosting, hydration, improved skin health, reduced risk for cancers, stimulated weight loss, prevention of osteoporosis, improved cardiometabolic health, and reduced blood pressure. However, there isn't enough evidence to support many of these health claims as being true.

What does science say about the alkaline water and diet?

Like many diets that are excessively popular and pitched to us through social media, there is more pseudoscientific support than actual scientific support for drinking alkaline waters or using an alkaline diet. While rodent studies offer some indication of benefit on the cellular level related to oxidative stress, there is not conclusive evidence to show the same for humans. The claim surrounding the impact on limiting cancer growth or preventing the development of cancers is based on the premise that cancer cells "thrive in acidic conditions" that is based on higher rates of anaerobic metabolism producing metabolic acids. Yet, the higher anaerobic metabolism stimulates blood vessel growth into the cancer development to adjust the delivery of materials into the cellular growth to minimize this acidic condition. Additionally, the assumption that consuming alkaline solutions will directly impact the pH of a specific region of the body is logically flawed. Moreover, there appears to be no or excessively limited evidence to support the claim that an alkaline diet or drinking alkaline water prevents cancer formation or reduces the growth of cancer cells if they have formed. Additionally, the regulation of pH is very tightly controlled by the body, and the excessive consumption of alkaline substances can easily disrupt this balance, cause gastrointestinal issues by disrupting normal stomach pH, and push the person into a condition referred to as alkalosis.

This takes us to the other forms of the liquid diet dogmas: the clear, full liquid or meal replacement liquid diet and the detox/cleansing liquid diet.

Liquid Diet

The idea of a liquid diet is to consume foods that have the potential to be liquid at room temperature or can be made into a liquid from their solid components. The liquid diet has been a hallmark of medical treatment for millennia, from teas and elixirs of antiquity to the cure-alls of the 1800s, 1900s, and even today; to the protein beverages used over the short term for treating various obesity and overfatness weight issues. The idea of liquid diets has not only spawned the cure-all beverages, but it is also the fundamental idea behind the smoothies and smoothie bars that rose to prominence in the late 1980s and early 1990s, along with mass-marketed "instant breakfast beverages" and dietary plans that have followers using meal replacement shakes instead of consuming meals. Not to mention the "vitamin and nutrient powders" advertised as the way to regain our health from the ravages of modern foods, or the "weight gainer" or "weight loss" protein shakes trumpeted by the self-proclaimed fitness experts across our social media feeds or jam-packed onto the shelves at the local store.

When looking at the various types of liquid diet, there is one diet that is typically advised by a medical professionals (i.e., doctor, nurse, nurse practitioner, or radiologist), the clear liquid diet. The clear liquid diet is typically advised to be followed for a few hours to a few days and generally in preparation for a medical imaging procedure or surgical procedure. Yet, followers of a clear liquid diet have extended this idea to go beyond this limited course of therapeutic treatment and into a general lifestyle of drinking "clear" liquids. What most people envision when the idea of "clear liquids" comes up is water, or a water diet, and yes, water is included in the beverages that can be consumed. But the idea of "clear" is referring to liquids not having added substances like milks, creams, or solid foods incorporated into the beverages being consumed; see Table Drink2.

Table Drink2. Examples of beverages and foods consumed following a liquid diet, based on the type of liquid diet

Clear Liquid	Full Liquid	Meal Replacement
Water, Sports drinks Electrolyte beverages, Soft drinks/Soda, Unsweetened Black Coffee, Black Tea, Green or Herbal Tea (without added dairy), Pulp less Fruit Juice or Fruit juice popsicles (without added dairy), Plain yogurts, Bone Broth (without solids), Jello or Gelatins (without solids), Honey, Syrups, Oils	Same as Clear Liquid along with: Coffee or Tea with dairy, Dairy beverages: Milk, Cream, Milkshakes without solids, Dairy Products: Ice Cream, Pudding, Sherbet, Yogurt, Frozen Yogurt without solids, Protein Shakes and fruit smoothies without solids, Creamed soups and porridge: Cream of Wheat, Cream of Ride, Tomato Soup, Creamed soups without solids Butters and Margarines, Soups or vegetable broths (without solids), Powdered nutritional beverages	Same list as full liquid, but at smaller quantities and with specific ingredients, and typically mass-produced and offered by mass-marketed company: Protein Shakes anc Smoothies (with or without solids) Powdered nutritional supplement beverages

Outside medical issues that indicate that a liquid diet is necessary, such as with enteral nutritional therapies (feeding tubes) or in the recovery process, what are the reasons given for following such a diet? The general premise that serves as the foundation for clear liquid diets is based on the idea that by extracting nutrients from foods, the liquids that are being consumed become healthier and more nutrient dense. That is, by "juicing" the foods that are being consumed, you are able to obtain the nutrition from the food without also having to ingest materials that the body does not need or that might disrupt our body's normal functions. An action that proponents claim to be true is that the time and effort put into the digestion of food becomes less, and the nutrients are ready to be absorbed as soon as they enter the mouth. There is also the indication that using a clear liquid diet that eliminates additional substances (i.e., sweeteners or artificial substances) from the diet while increasing vitamin, mineral, and antioxidant intake, the diet can act to "detoxify" the body. Additionally, when proponents of the clear liquid diet fall back onto the misguided notion of the Caloric balance, they claim that by removing dairy and sweeteners from the beverages, there are fewer Calories in the diet and it will not only help to make you healthier but also promote weight loss, too.

Table Drink3. Purported benefits coming from a liquid diet that are cited by followers as a reason for using the liquid diets.

Weight Loss	Increased Hydration
Retention of Fat-Free Mass	Detoxification Effect
Weight Gain	Improved Digestion and Nutrition
Increased Satiety	Improved Brain Functions and Alertness
Bone Growth	Improved cardiometabolic health
Muscle Growth	Improved immune functions
Reduced inflammation	Reduced Blood Pressure

Claims that are extended to the other forms of the liquid diet even though each has additional items that are allowed in the diet from what is consumed by followers of the clear liquid diet, table Drink3. The proponents of the full liquid and meal-replacement forms of the liquid diet state their form of the liquid diet is better than the clear liquid diet as it allows for beverages to contain mixtures within them, as long as solids are not generally present in the beverages. The full liquid and meal replacement liquid diets are also the forms of the liquid diets that we tend to be more familiar with and are seen throughout advertisements for "health" drinks, "weight loss" or "weight gainer" protein drinks, or the mass-marketed powders that fill many of our social media feeds (e.g., AG-1, Huel, SlimFast, Balance Nutrition, Boost Nutrition, Ka' Chava). A caveat that proponents fall back on when discussing the easiness of following the diets and how the options make it more appealing to them as followers of the tenets of the diet. There are also the claims from the companies that produce the ready-made products or shops that produce the beverages (e.g., smoothie bars, nutrition stores, coffee shops) that stipulate the diet becomes more nutritious because their powders and beverages have a higher density relative to what can be consumed from either the whole food alternative or what might be available from the beverages of the clear liquid diet. Additionally, we get claims that by utilizing meal-replacement liquids and beverages, the older followers of this dogmatic dietary practice are able to increase their nutrient load and offset any adverse effects that aging has on the ability to maintain fat-free mass (e.g., skeletal muscle, bone, skin) that might otherwise be lost.

What does science say about liquid diets?

A lot of the claims that are offered by proponents of the liquid diet dogmas and the mass marketers follow many pseudoscientific principles where claims stem from hasty overgeneralizations of limited research or use cherry-picked results of benefit. This is where a caveat needs to be addressed: most of the research that has been offered related to liquid diets falls into one of three avenues: weight loss focused on overfatness and diabetic management, athlete dietary supplementation, and those attempting the stop muscle wasting (as seen in older people, those undergoing cancer treatment, or those suffering from AIDS). From these three avenues of research, we have extrapolated a lot of information to generalize for the entire human population, but to be accurate, let's focus specifically on what is being stated from each.

For those using the liquid diets for both weight loss or improving diabetic condition, there is ample evidence that any form of the liquid diet is effective for short-term weight loss, reduced fat mass, and improved cardiometabolic health. With greater effectiveness when the liquid diet uses higher protein and lower carbohydrates in the total nutrient load being consumed, with most reports based on the misguided notion of Calories and not the requisite nutrients, greater benefits are seen when Calories are kept constant but nutrients are altered. The rationalization that is offered parallels other diets that report benefits in body weight, body composition, or cardiometabolic health; changes in nutrition and the metabolites available lead to alterations in glucose and fat metabolism. These changes reduce glucose in the blood and improve the actions of Insulin, Glucagon and Leptin at regulating metabolism and feelings of being full or hungry. Along with this change, there is an increase in the use of fat for fuel leading to a greater amount of fats being broken down in adipose tissues (fat cells) that changes fat cell hormones being released, improving metabolic functions and reduce inflammation signals. When coupled with reduced carbohydrates in the diet, there is an increase in ketogenesis (making ketones) that, with the improved use of fats for fuels and normalizing glucose metabolism, reduces oxidative stress in the body related to energy metabolism that further reduces inflammation and helps to improve immune functions. At the liver, there is a change in fat and cholesterol metabolism that leads to a reduction in total cholesterol and low-density lipoproteins (LDL) that are found circulating in the blood. The last change in cardiometabolic health is associated with a high-protein liquid diet where there is a change in cortisol release and converting enzymes that generate cortisol from other steroid hormones at the tissues of the body, allowing for retention of proteins in the fat-free mass of the body. A key component in ensuring that during periods of weight loss, fat-free mass is retained while fat mass is lost.

At the same time, those following the liquid diet for weight loss, when the nutrients in the liquids are severely restricted, as measured in published research by Calories, the ability to cause weight loss becomes minimized. While weight loss will occur, the rate and total amount of weight loss are going to be less in the severely restricted dieters versus those that are using a less restricted form of the liquid diet. There are also noted decreases in the performance of the body in several functional areas (most noted loss of strength, endurance, and mental acuity) when the diet is severely restricted. The ability for one to self-select to follow the liquid diets over longer durations becomes lower when the choice of foods or amount of nutrients that can be consumed as liquids are severely restricted, due to the loss of positive reinforcements that the choice has for someone. This is why most research indicates using the highly restricted liquid diets for only a few days and up to 4 weeks at most, with some speculation being offered that cycling between restricted and less restrictive versions of the liquid diets might be beneficial for followers to use as weight loss and maintenance is the reason for choosing to follow this dogmatic diet.

On the opposite side of the coin to weight loss are those that use the full liquid and meal replacement liquid diet to assist in gaining weight. This line of evidence is coming from the athletic and exercising populations and comes into play, and there is a secondary caveat that must be addressed. There is no evidence that independent of exercise there is a benefit to the skeletal muscle or bones in terms of growth or improvement in the health of the tissue. With that caveat out of the way, there is ample evidence that using high-protein, high-carbohydrate meal replacement beverages and liquid diet principles has beneficial effects on the growth seen in skeletal muscle, bones, and connective tissues (e.g., ligaments and tendons) following exercise. The responses seen are greatest when exercise is lower than what would typically be used for promoting muscle growth, such as when focusing on endurance training, or when performing maximal effort with minimal training volume (sets and repetitions) that would provide the duration of exercise necessary to stimulate growth. The rationale given for the benefits to athletes or exercisers comes from providing a positive nutrient balance, especially if carbohydrate load is around the 10-12 g/kg (or 4.5-5.4 g/lbs) of body mass and an amino acid or nitrogen balance is nearing 3.0 g/kg (or 1.36 g/lbs) of body mass. The positive nitrogen balance is associated with amino acid availability that helps to promote and support protein building during the recovery from exercise, while the positive carbohydrate balance ensures that fuel sources are maintained and that glycogen and protein are not being broken in order to meet the needs of the body for fuel to generate the ATP necessary for work to be completed.

The other group that shows a weight gain effect is those attempting to prevent muscle wasting (excessive weight loss due to age or disease). In this group, the use of the liquid diet allows for a nutrition balance to be achieved, and when a high -protein liquid diet is followed there is a reduction in cortisol signals that help regulate inflammation but also help to block cortisol's effect on breaking down fat-free tissues (i.e., skeletal muscle, bone). This action helps to slow down the speed that wasting occurs at, and when coupled with a positive nutrient balance, can help to reverse the wasting.

Detox or Cleansing Diet

A large swath of proponents of the liquid diet not only tout the ability to encourage weight loss or weight gain, depending on goals, but also the implicit ability to allow the body to "cleanse" itself from toxins. There is some indication that liquid diets containing fruit and vegetable extracts can provide micronutrients (i.e., phytochemicals, vitamins, coenzymes, and minerals) that can assist with controlling oxidative stress. The ability to control oxidative stress can reduce inflammation and immune activity and can assist cells in the liver and kidney to perform chemical reactions to eliminate molecules that might interfere with metabolism that could possibly have a toxic effect on our health.

An idea that takes us into the next diet dogma within the liquid diet practices, the detox or cleansing diets.

Let's start with a quick review of terms here. A toxin is a chemical or molecule that has the potential to disrupt metabolism and cause adverse effects on health. While a poison is a toxic chemical that stops or interferes with metabolism, and at specific amounts or for specific amounts of time, can kill someone, not just cause adverse effects on health. Any chemical or molecule that we consume (even those things in a "detox" solution) has the potential to be a toxin based on two key features: dose and duration. A dose is the amount of a substance; in order to have a dose response, the molecule must be in a form that is referred to as bioactive (able to interact with cells). Duration is how long the substance is present, the duration of exposure is going to be inversely dependent on the dose that is necessary to be toxic, where the more toxic a substance is, the shorter the duration to reach a point of being a toxin, and it gets reversed for substances that are less toxic.

Based on the idea that toxins are being consumed or are circulating throughout our body, there arises specific dogmatic diets meant to eliminate these toxins, a detox diet. These dogmatic dietary practices usually involve restricting what is consumed, either food or beverage, over the course of a few days, a few weeks, or even a few months, or using the hallmark of the detox diet drinking specific beverages (e.g., teas, juices, broths, water with added nutrients) over the eating of foods with the exception of specific fruits and vegetables, or dietary supplements and herbs; see Table Drink4.

The tenets of the detox diet are centered on the basis that chemicals are easily divided into "good chemicals" and "bad chemicals" without acknowledging that when looking into toxicity, the dose of the chemical and the length of exposure are the real determinants of what is "good" or what is "bad" as it relates to the chemicals in our diet. From the perspective of the proponents of the diet, the detox drinks, along with fruits, vegetables, supplements, and herbs, will work because they fall into one of three primary chemical categories. The active substance functions as an antioxidant chemical that removes oxidative species or as a laxative to help with removal of feces from the intestines.

Marketing of the detox diets is commonly seen as "cleanses" with the impetus that you need to cleanse or "clean" your digestive system of toxins or fecal matter. Proponents of the detox diets claim that following the diet lets the body rid itself of toxins, e.g., heavy metals and chemicals from food or the environment, that impair your body from functioning appropriately. The other thing that proponents claim that the detox diet does is help someone lose weight, in particular "intestinal weight" or "water weight," but it will also encourage fat loss. The claim is that by focusing on drinking the detox elixirs while avoiding food, you are able to improve overall health and lose weight at the same time.

Table Drink4. Chemicals, foods, and supplements that are regularly used by followers of the detox diet based on the proponents indicating each having a detoxifying effect on the body

Foods	Chemicals and Supplements

Vegetables:
    Artichoke, Asparagus, Avocado, Beets, Broccoli, Brussels Sprout, Cauliflower, Cabbage, Carrot, Celery, Collard Greens, Cucumbers, Endives, Garlic, Grapefruit, Jicama, Kelp, Leeks, Lettuce, Okra, Onions, Radishes, Rutabaga, Snow Peas, Spinach, Sweet Potatoes, Squash
Fruits:
    Acai, Apples, Apricots, Blackberries, Blueberries, Cantaloupe, Cherries, Cranberries, Grapefruit, Figs, Grapes, Guava, Kiwi, Lemon, Lime, Loganberries, Mango, Nectarines, Oranges, Papaya, Peaches, Pears, Pineapple, Plums, Pomegranate, Prunes, Raspberries, Strawberries, Tangerines, Watermelon Beans and Legumes: Peas (Split and Yellow), Lentils, Black Beans, Black-Eyed Peas, Kidney Beans, Lima
	Drinks:
	    Herbal Teas, Lemon Waters, Fermented Beverages (Kombucha), Infused Water
	Vitamins, Cofactors and provitamins::
	    Vitamin A, Vitamin B_1, Vitamin B_6, Vitamin C, Vitamin E, Vitamin K, Riboflavin, Flavonoids, Beta-carotene

Grains, Nuts and Seeds (or their oils):	Herbs and Supplements:
Almonds, Arrowroot, Barley, Brazil Nuts, Buckwheat, Chia, Coconut, Flax Seeds, Hemp Seeds, Millet, Pistachios, Poppy Seeds, Pumpkin Seeds, Sunflower Seeds, Walnuts	Dandelion, Garlic, Milk thistle, Rosemary, Schizandra, Turmeric Supplements: Activated Charcoal, N-Acetylcysteine, Probiotics, Psyllium, Resveratrol, Spirulina

The claims serve as the basis for why followers sell the detox diets to others, including:

- The promise of purification through toxin elimination that is connected with a sense that there is contamination within the body based on what we are being exposed to
- Thinking about food and drinks gives a sense of control over internal processes that are largely out of our control
- Perform a cyclic relationship of making conscious choices of inclusion and exclusion, of "cleansing" that can allow for having health needs met

What does science say about detox diets?

Based on the anatomy of the human body, the physiology of specific organs (i.e., liver, lungs, sweat glands and sebaceous glands of the skin, and kidneys) there is actually no reason for a detoxification diet. Each of the organs listed is able to excrete metabolic wastes and toxins from the body, and the liver and kidney are able to perform chemical reactions that are able to make active chemicals inactive and "detoxify" the blood of metabolites that might be considered a toxin, chemicals that would disrupt the function of the cells of the body. There is some evidence that addition of antioxidants and co-enzyme metabolites from our diet can have an impact on the effectiveness of the liver to perform the reactions necessary to "detoxify" or turn a bioactive molecule into a biologically inert molecule. However, this is not an indication that the detox diets themselves are the cause for the improved effectiveness being seen in the ability for liver cells to perform the reactions. From this perspective, those that are skeptical of the detox diet's dogmatic tenets stipulate that not only are detox diets unnecessary, but they can also be harmful to the followers of this diet, leading to malnourishment, nutrient deficiency, or even the possible overdosing on certain supplements (that can be toxic or poisonous to the person and defeats the rationale for following such a diet).

What can we say about liquid diets, detox diets, or the alkaline water diets?

When looking at the liquid diets, there are various health and weight loss claims that are supported in the case of medical care. However, outside the healthcare setting, the claims are not as supported as within the healthcare setting. When compared to equal nutrient load, there appears to be no difference relative to claims of weight loss or weight gain, antioxidant delivery, or rate of recovery. As far as the alkaline water and detox diets go, the popularity and general adherence often come from large and grandiose claims about what each can do (e.g., allow you to lose weight quickly, prevent cancers from growing or spreading, and cleanse your body through the removal of "harmful" substances). But it is very important to recognize that the evidence we have from rigorous and unbiased scientific studies states that neither are able to live up to the promises. More importantly, each can be very dangerous for overall health if used for prolonged periods of time.

Pros
- Short-term weight loss with maintenance of fat-free mass during weight loss
- Potential for stimulating effect to promote muscle growth at suboptimal levels of training intensity and can be used to ensure that protein and nitrogen balance is met
- Short-term reduction in inflammation and improved liver and immune functions due to antioxidant availability
- Improved cardiometabolic health (improved cholesterol levels with reduced LDL levels, improved glucose metabolism with normalization of Insulin, Glucagon, Leptin) and reduced blood pressure due to the effect of increased nitrous oxide and BCAA on blood vessel functions

Cons
- Potential to lead to malnourishment that is associated with rapid weight loss attributed to the various liquid diets or to detox diets

- Potential to be exposed to metabolic or endocrine disruptors that can lead to issues of overfatness and compromised cardiometabolic health
- Propagates misinformation about diet and foods that has the potential to exacerbate food aversions and disordered eating behaviors
- Potentially harmful metabolic conditions and reduced microbiome diversity based on changes in pH within the digestive system

Take-home message

Under certain conditions and based on various scenarios, a liquid diet can be of benefit. The use of protein-based beverages as meal replacements or in the aid of weight loss has been shown to be safe and effective. The use of whey protein drink have been shown to be effective in reducing blood vessel inflammation when combined with other diet and exercise modifications to treat heart disease. The use of liquid diets is a staple of inpatient medical care and for those that are undergoing surgical procedures where it is recommended to avoid solid foods. Meaning that, for certain individuals and in certain circumstances, the use of liquid diets may be beneficial to either increase nutrient intake or serve as the only means by which nutrition can be achieved

For those that are attempting to gain muscle mass, bone mass, and strength through exercise, protein supplement beverages can provide added amino acids and nitrogen necessary for building muscle and bone. But there is no indication that using expensive ultraprocessed and refined protein powders gives a greater benefit relative to the less expensive protein blends..

However, the tenets held for why to use some of the liquid diets tend to perpetuate unhealthy relationships with food and nourishment. Perpetuation of misguided notions about having "good" and "bad" foods or that body weight and body composition are somehow the result of the Calories in the foods that we are eating. Misguided notions and misrepresentation of information that for some can lead to dangerous eating behaviors and even food avoidance.

I am one with my food and my food is one with me...

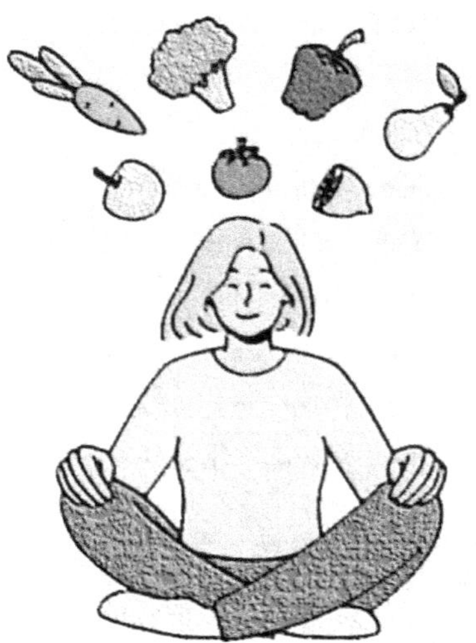

A lot of the dogmatic diets come about through the acceptance that diets can have a curative value to them. In the case of some diets, that curative value is being able to reduce body weight. This leads the discussion to a host of diets that I like to think of as our "centering" diets. Diets, eating styles, and lifestyles that are built off of a diet are meant to teach us portion control and to be aware of the how, what, when, and why we are eating. Philosophical tenets that, in the end, are meant to be used to ultimately control how much we eat. Messaging that starts with proportionality diets (see *Calories go in...*) but goes beyond to look at how to change the proportions of food we eat without severely limiting or eliminating any specific macronutrient for the diet. These diets are the bulk of diets that we see being marketed to us, provide us with the prepared meals necessary to fit into our busy lives, and teach us the "dos" and "don'ts" of how to eat and when to eat. So, let's take a look at the diet dogmas that would help explain why people follow the plans offered by Mindful Eating, Knives over Forks, NOOM, Full Plate, Jenny Craig, Weight Watchers, Factor, Nutrisystem, or HelloFresh, just to name a few.

The general tenet across all of these different marketed diets is that if you follow our guide and eat our specialized food, you will not only feel better but you will also lose weight at the same time. But the interesting thing is that all of them purport that theirs is the simplest and truest way to reach that goal, even when offering the exact same central idea... eat less, less "bad food," less "fatty food," and less "processed" foods (even while selling processed foods). The sales pitch being offered by any of the proponents for any of the diets is that by following this tenet you begin to understand portion size, understand "good" versus "bad" when it comes to food, and learn how to cook to eliminate fast food from your diet. Because your excess weight is coming from overeating, from having too much "bad" food, and especially because of eating any amount of fast food.

Mindful Eating: from Mindfulness to Knives over Forks and NOOM

Mindfulness is not a new phenomenon with its roots in many ancient religious practices that teach you to be present in the moment. The idea of mindful eating stems from this idea as part of the holistic stress management program developed in the 1970s that started out to not primarily focus on either health or weight loss outcomes, like many of the other dogmatic diets like to preach about. With the original application paying little focus to Calories, carbohydrates, fats, proteins, or any of the other hot-button issues that foment many conversations we have on diets and dieting... but over the last few decades the idea of mindful eating has become a stable component of diet programs that focus on these specific aspects of food and can be considered central to the philosophy of the Knives over Forks and the NOOM diet programs and several other diet applications designed for the smart devices that govern our modern lives. Whether one follows the original tenet of mindfulness or the modern applications in dietary programs meant for weight loss or improved health, mindful eating focuses on the dogma that followers need to pay attention to their food without judgment. An approach to food that focuses on sensual (i.e., taste, smell, texture) awareness of the food and the experience the food elicits to the psyche during and after a meal while staying in the moment. Through this approach, you become more aware of not only what you are eating but also why you might be eating and how much you are eating.

Based on the tenet of awareness and staying in the moment, proponents of mindful eating have the ability to help with weight loss and becoming healthy, even though that is not the primary focus. As they insist, the eating style that encourages you to stay in the moment allows you to savor the food and the eating experience by slowing the rate that you are eating. By bringing full awareness to each plate, or bite, of food from the first thought about food to the last bite without focusing on the consequences of the experience but on the experience of eating itself, it provides reinforcement to what an appropriate portion of food might be, but more importantly discourages negative reinforcers or avoidance of food that are commonly associated with eating issues or overfatness. Proponents of the diet use this awareness and eating style to support their assertion that mindful eating leads to eating less, and by eating less, leads to weight loss.

Followers of mindful eating have a sense of who they are by following 6 general attitudes and principles around eating:

1. Listen to the signals that the body is sending to tell you when you are full while eating.

2. Understand the signals for when you are actually hungry versus bored or in response to adverse emotions.
3. Be mindful about how you arrange your kitchen so that everything is purposefully placed to encourage appropriate eating behaviors and discourage scavenging for food to eliminate mindless eating.
4. Understand the motivations you have for food; don't indulge or seek comfort with food that you are eating, but be mindful of what the food is and what the food will become for you.
5. Connect with your food, understand where it originated and what it will allow you to do because of the nutrients that you are consuming, show gratitude for having the food, the traditions around meals, and the people you are eating with.
6. Attend to your meal, not to everything else that might be happening outside of the meal. Limit multitasking and distractions around meals; establish mealtimes where you have to slow down and use a specific area (i.e., kitchen table) to sit down at when you eat.

Mindful eating develops a nonjudgmental and self-accepting way to eat and to develop your diet that encourages appreciation of food rather than restricting specific macronutrients or excessively restricting food altogether. By being fully aware of your food, it encourages followers to trust that they are making the best decisions rather than entrenching them with restrictions and rules about what to eat, how to eat, or when to eat. You might be thinking, OK, this sounds kind of kooky, but there has to be a reason for using this dieting style, right?

What benefits might be achieved from Mindful Eating?

Most of the benefits related to body and metabolic health that arise from mindful eating are going to be associated with limiting overeating. By controlling triggers for overeating, those who are overweight can establish positive reinforcers to encourage lifestyle changes and the resulting improvements in body weight, body composition, and overall health. While these are indirect benefits, there are some direct benefits that proponents offer for why one should follow a mindful eating diet. These include increased awareness of hunger and fullness, limiting emotional eating, a reduction of stress and negative thoughts about food, a reduction in binge eating and overeating, generating healthier food choices, and an increased satisfaction with foods and choices of meals.

This sounds a little too good; *what about risks and costs?*

All of the diet dogmas appear to have risks and costs involved with them. Unlike a lot of the other dogmatic diets, there are not really any inherent risks of deficiencies, as long as you are making appropriate food choices to meet your nutrient needs. There could be a cost for those that are not highly organized and have the ability to schedule meals and mealtimes to allow for mindful eating practices, but with better organization and time management these costs can be overcome.

What does the science say?

There is speculation within the literature that mindful eating can be effective at reducing eating disorder-like behaviors and stress that surrounds food choices and meals for those that are attempting to diet to lose weight. There are some clinical observations that mindful eating can be beneficial in the nutrition aspect of treatment for non-communicable diseases. Along with evidence to support its use in general weight loss programs, it has also been shown to be effective in teaching portion sizes and reinforcement of appropriate portion sizes for those that are frequent consumers of fast food and pre-packaged foods where portions are regularly exaggerated. Outside of general eating behaviors, there is evidence that mindful eating has positive effects on digestive functions, and by slowing down how quickly one eats, it reduces the symptoms of digestive distress (i.e., GERD, acid reflux, irritable bowel) that may be exhibited.

What can we say about mindful eating?

The mindful eating approach is a useful and common-sense approach to eating that leads to eating less, having lower food anxiety, and a better sense of what nutrients are needed for the person. The practice of mindful eating can lessen the likelihood of developing eating disorders in people who are susceptible to those issues. It is an approach that can be integrated into any of the other dogmatic diets quite easily and is readily associated with the other diets discussed in this section to reduce total food intake in an effective medically supervised weight loss program.

Pros
- Highly flexible, and not restrictive, that allows for easy use.
- Promotes behavioral changes related to meals and eating that reduce food anxiety and negative thoughts about foods or meals
- Not restrictive, there are few to no food rules with mindful eating, with some programs offering advice on selection for foods that offer better nutrients relative to other foods, but there is no indication for "good" or "bad" foods or foods that need to be eliminated
- Very low chance of having any nutrient deficiencies developing while following mindful eating
- Encourages weight loss and improvement in overall health through appropriate food choices and slowing down eating to ultimately eat less, with food that is more in line with nutrient needs for the body.

Cons
- Time-consuming process with each meal and the need to dedicate specific times of the day to eating
- May need to alter entire lifestyle around meal prep and mealtime to ensure that you are practicing mindfulness through the entire process
- May have unforeseen costs to any of the smart-device programs or NOOM programs that can be limiting to practices for long periods of time
- If the desire of following tenets is weight loss, the outcome of using mindfulness and mindful eating may not match and could be discouraging to the follower.

Full Plate Living, Mass-marketed Lifestyle Plans

The other style of dieting and lifestyle modification that resides within the confines of the "centering" are the diet plans and lifestyle that focus on two aspects of lifestyle meant to influence changes in body weight and overall health. The first is to change portions and proportions of macronutrients in the diet while also promoting other changes in lifestyle through the development of a supportive community. The development comes via either open marketing and community activities or through a sense of being part of a community that allows you to be integrated into something larger than oneself.

The general tenets that are being offered, whether you follow Full Plate Living, Weight Watchers, Jenny Craig, or any of the other mass-marketed lifestyles, are that by making small changes in the macronutrients (namely swapping fiber-poor foods in your diet for fiber-rich foods), using support networks and sponsors, and increasing levels of physical activity, you are able to lose weight and become healthier. Ostensibly, the dogma of the diet is one based around moderation with the assertion that what they offer is not a fad diet with achievable goals that can be obtained only through their distinct program, even when they are not exactly unique.

All of the components of these lifestyle diets center on two major propositions. First, add fiber to their diet and limit portions of food eaten at each meal. Second, add beverages to meals and between meals that offer limited nutrients but increase satiety (i.e., water, teas, coffees). While lifestyle modification typically comes from helpful and common-sense advice that is accompanied by a collection of tools and support networks that make weight loss and health improvement attainable through small lifestyle changes that are adaptable to our modern lifestyle. The idea is to provide the tools, knowledge, and support necessary to make the process of changing one's lifestyle enjoyable while reinforcing that benefits may not be seen quickly but the benefits are potentially enormous when followed for a long-period.

When separating these dogmas out into subclasses, we start noticing slight differences in the points of emphasis in following these central tenets. For those that follow the model of Full Plate Living, we can break the difference into two points of emphasis: increase the fruit and vegetable portion of each meal to increase overall daily fiber intake and reduce (or avoid) processed and mass-produced foods that have made an ever-growing percentage of food we consume. The idea is that by following this point of emphasis, the disciples of the diet are able to offset or reverse the metabolic issues that arise from eating processed foods or foods high in fat and refined sugars (i.e., metabolic syndrome, cardiovascular disease). While the followers of the other mass-marketed lifestyle interventions insist their key points of emphasis are to eat less total food, eat less processed foods (unless that processed food comes from us), reduce sugar intake, increase fiber intake when choosing fruits, vegetables, or grains, and increase physical activity and exercise. With a few of these dogmatic programs adding to their repertoire the use of weight tracking and group meetings to support the followers in their weight loss journey and hopefully weight maintenance.

What are the benefits that can be seen?

Proponents of all of the diets here claim that following the diet leads to weight loss. Weight loss comes about through the changing proportion of food groups being consumed or through the misguided notion of reducing Caloric intake to cause weight loss.

Those that follow the Full Plate methods also report that following the diet leads to improvements in cardiometabolic health by lowering total cholesterol and LDL levels, normalizing glucose levels and reducing inflammation. Changes that they state reduce the risk for cardiovascular disease, along with altering metabolism that leads to changes in mental awareness. Additionally, they stipulate that following the diet leads to improvement in subjective sense of stamina, and reduce the sense of fatigue, allow for better sleep, and overtime leads to improvement in digestive functions and the microbiome of the intestines. As to the last point here, proponents of the diet argue that by changing the microbiome, the diet will have a long-lasting impact on improved overall health independent of changes in the weight.

As for the other cluster of diets, the proponents tout the ability to learn portion size and balances in food group proportions in the diet. Most will use ready-to-eat meals or specific recipes that the followers are able to cook at home. A secondary benefit that is touted as coming from the diet dogma is learning how to plan your meals, prep and cook meals at home that combine to limit the need to eat fast food or processed foods. Outside of learning about food and food portions, cooking and preparing meals, the proponents of following the mass-marketed diet lifestyles stipulate that on top of weight loss, the various diets can be used to reduce indices of diabetes (i.e., high blood sugar, poor Insulin sensitivity, elevated A1c levels). There are also statements from followers of the diet that it improves cardiovascular health by reducing cholesterol and triglyceride levels in the blood along with a reduction in blood pressure. There is also indication that food anxiety can be reduced during and after use of the diets primarily through the use of planned meals or establishing a meal plan.

What are the risks and costs for using these diets?

For all of the diets here, there are costs and risks that need to be considered. The biggest is the actual economic cost that using these plans might have for the follower. All dietary dogmas in this category involve purchasing books and online resources, buying into a meal service program, paying monthly fees, or a combination of all of these that can be burdensome for some to follow the plans for long periods.

There is also an increase in consuming plant-based foods, which means that based on how much the proportions have shifted, there could be anti-nutrient issues that parallel what vegans and vegetarians might face (see *Go Green*). Along with a possible imbalance in the ratio of omega-3 to omega-6 fatty acids in the diet, in favor of the omega-6 fatty acids, that might lead to increases in inflammation instead of the reduced inflammation that is claimed to be one of the benefits here.

When looking at programs like Weight Watchers that use public meetings that may involve discussion of body weight and weight changes, there can be a negative reinforcement to the plan based on what the scale is recording. The reliance on such public discussions of weight can lead to aversion and eating issues possibly developing in order to reach goals that have been established. Metabolically, because of the restriction in total nutrient intake, there can be a negative hormonal response that might adversely impact the ability to get the body weight or body composition changes that can be sought. With the use of pre-packaged and processed foods, there is a risk of consuming metabolic disruptors that can impact the ability to achieve the benefits that are indicated as coming from the diet and lifestyles.

What does the science say about these diets?

Most of the research into these diet dogmas focuses on weight loss, weight maintenance, or reversal of metabolic syndrome issues (e.g., Type-2 Diabetes, cardiovascular disease), and in the case of mindful eating as a way to control food anxiety.

Looking into these diets as a means to promote weight loss and weight maintenance, the consensus among available studies is that these are effective dietary plans. There is no evidence to indicate that one style is more effective than any other style within this cluster of dogmatic diets. There is also evidence that suggested the use of dogmas like Full Plate Living or programmed diets like Weight Watchers, Jenny Craig, or others is an effective way to improve cardiometabolic health while reducing body weight and shifting body composition. Improvements that are speculated but not definitively linked with the changes in fat cell hormones that lead to normalization of inflammation signals and improvements in glucose metabolism and increases in responsiveness to Insulin, GLP-1, and Leptin. Of the evidence that we have, there is greater support for the use of Full Plate and Weight Watchers than the other dietary and lifestyle programs, but this might be due to report issues more than the effectiveness of any single dietary program.

Psychologists have also indicated agreement that it can lead to a reduction of food cravings, with improved awareness of portion control and a need to be more physically active in order to cause the change in body weight that is desired within the treatment. Public health advocates have noted that the practices associated with Full Plate Living have reduced feelings of food insecurity while also reducing the reliance on pre-packaged and processed foods for meals or snacks. In conjunction with other lifestyle treatments for metabolic issues associated with overfatness, mindful eating has been shown to be an effective way to improve diabetic indices that appear to parallel a reduction in fat mass that the public health research has speculated at but not definitively shown to be form reduction of the pro-inflammatory hormones that are seen in overfatness. There is, however, evidence from these studies to indicate a reduction in stress that is seen with a mindful approach to life and eating leading to a normalization to inflammation and stress hormones. Changes that help to explain how mindful eating can increase sensitivity to Insulin, GLP-1, and Leptin that helps to reverse the signs and symptoms of metabolic syndrome and possible diabetes.

What can be said about these diets?

The use of lifestyle diets and programs is an effective and easy method to learn about food portions and how to control portions of food being eaten. For those that have limited experience cooking, the use of planned meals, recipes, or pre-packed ingredients for meals can teach food prep and cooking skills necessary to reduce the consumption of processed pre-packaged foods. These dogmatic approaches increase personal and community responsibilities through the development of support networks that help to reinforce goals and aims for the individual person. There is a wide variety of foods and food choices that make the dietary programs excessively flexible and unique for the individual that encourages experimentation that keeps experiences novel and unique to encourage continuation in following the tenets of the dietary and lifestyle plans.

Pros

- Diets are generally easy to follow with convenient tools and guides for preparing meals to align with dogmatic principles without requiring specific foods to be eaten or macronutrients to be included or excluded from the diet.
- Offers a sense of community to the followers with a vast support network to rely on.
- Promotes "healthy" eating and lifestyle over either weight loss or improving overall health, even if these happen with the change in eating and lifestyle.

Cons

- Potential negative reinforcer or psychological punishment that can accompany using the scale to measure responses and results along with avoidance that can come from public awareness of body weight and body weight changes.
- Potential to be socially exclusionary for individuals who wish to eat at restaurants or socialize with others outside of the dietary group around meals
- Economic costs to using the programs; you have to pay to follow the diet, and costs can be an exclusionary factor.

Take-home message

Most of the advice offered through the "centering" diets are simple, easy, and generally considered to be common sense in the approach. There are no specific macronutrients (i.e., carbohydrates, lipids, proteins) that someone following the diet is to restrict or exclude, which makes these dietary dogmas very flexible. When looking at the application of the tenets preached by the followers, the popular use of the "centering" diets comes from the desire to reverse the pandemic of overfatness that has been on the rise for the last half-century. A rise that is typically associated with excessive consumption of mass-produced ultra-processed foods. The "centering" diets allow one to focus on why, how, and when they are eating.

Through the practices preached by diets like mindful eating, NOOM, Full Plate Living, Weight Watchers, Jenny Craig, Hello Fresh, Nutrisystem, that someone is able to reduce food cravings while learning portion control and proportionality of food groups within the diet that are necessary for maintaining or changing body weight and body composition. The tenets that are preached here have become the hallmark of many medically supervised "low-calorie diet" programs that are meant to not only cause weight loss but also teach portion size and reduce total food intake in an effort to allow for long-term weight loss and subsequent weight maintenance.

Curiouser and Curiouser...

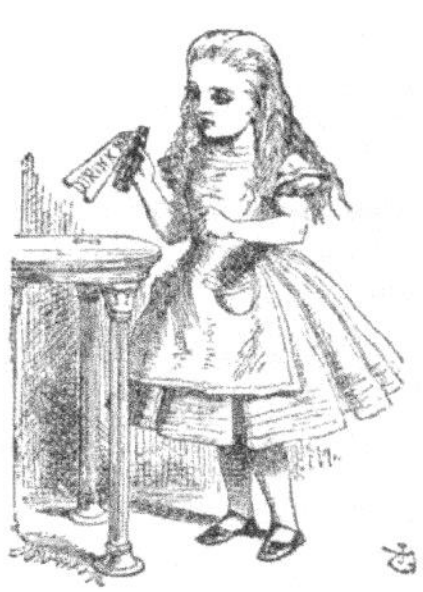

"Well, I'll eat it," said Alice, "and if it makes me grow larger, I can reach the key; and if it makes me grow smaller, I can creep under the door..." *– Alice,*
Alice in Wonderland*, Lewis Carroll*

We now reach the point in our discussion of the more peculiar dietary dogmas that buttress the modern era of fad diets (i.e., the HCG diet, macrobiotic diets) that have come into vogue over the last decade. Fad diets that appear to be nothing more than rebrands of the many dogmatic diets that have been discussed here that gained popularity in the last half-century and especially after the start of the 21st century. The stipulation of what I like to think of as the curious diet dogmas is that not only are there "good" foods and "bad" foods, but the difference is both individualized and generalized at the same time. Some of these dogmatic ideals about diets are based on pseudoscientific explanations and a belief system that diets are able to be tailored to the person due to their unique characteristics, yet they are still generalizable to allow anyone to follow the diet.

And what are these curious dietary dogmas? The bland-food diet. The blood-type diet. The gluten-free diet. While diets like the gluten-free diet are based on the dietary treatment of digestive illness. And, if you listen to how people discuss food, it seems as if everyone has that digestive illness. The other diets are formed from pseudoscientific principles regarding human anatomy and physiology rather than medical treatment for a specific condition.

Bland Food Diets

The bland diet, sometimes referred to as a "low residue diet" or "soft diet," was developed originally as a dietary practice for treatment for people that suffer from issues within their digestive system (i.e., reflux, irritable bowel). An idea that has been extended beyond this small population to be usable by everyone with the central tenet is to eat foods strictly to obtain the nutrients contained within the food. Where the foods that are allowed within the diet need to be both easy to digest and limit the bliss response that comes from eating foods. This means choosing foods that are typically easy to chew, low in fat, low in fiber, and mildly spiced to non-spiced, table Curious1. Additionally, proponents of following the bland diet, insist that not only are you avoiding spicy, fried, or raw foods, but also avoiding alcohol or caffeinated beverages. The origin of the bland diet has its roots throughout medical history with it rising to prominence as a recognized dietary practice in the mid 1900s.

A bland food diet is generally followed by individuals that experience digestive issues from eating spicy foods or have symptoms of digestive system diseases or distress. The general idea of the diet is to provide foods that are easy to digest and is not a diet that is specific to either allowing for weight loss, maintenance, or to improve health for the person beyond digestive issues. A bland diet may be prescribed by a healthcare provider as part of treatment for non-communicable disease, but in an effort to provide nutrients not as a curative.

Table Curious1. Summary of foods that are often included or excluded within the Bland Food Diet.

Vegetables	Fruits (or Juices)	Dairy

Include:
  Beets
  Carrots
  Green Beans
  Peas
  Potatoes
  Spinach
  Pumpkin
	Include:
	  Avocado
	  Banana
	  Melons
		Include:
		  Low-fat Animal-derived milk
		  Yogurt
		  Mild Cheeses (American, Cottage, Cheddar)
		  Low-fat Ice creams

Exclude:
  Cabbage
  Cruciferous (Brussels Sprouts, Broccoli, Cauliflower)
  Onion
  Garlic
  Lentils
  Legumes (Beans, Soybeans)
  Peppers
  Tomato
	Exclude:
	  Berries (Blackberry, Blueberry, Cranberry, Raspberry, Strawberry)
	  Citrus (Oranges, Lemons, Limes, Grapefruits)
	  Grapes
	  Dried Fruits (Prunes, Raisins)
		Exclude:
		  Plant-based beverages
		  Non-dairy Ice-cream, cheese, butter
		  Whole milk
		  Heavy cream
		  Ice cream
		  Soft cheeses (Blue Cheese, Brie, Monterey Jack, Roquefort)

Nuts and Seeds (including oils and butters)	**Meats and Alternatives**	**Grains and Cereals**

Include:
  Refined nut and seed oils
  Refined nut butters
	Include:
	  Eggs
	  Chicken (skinless, white meat)
	  Shellfish (Crab, Crayfish, Lobster, Prawn, Shrimp)
	  Silken Tofu
		Include:
		  Oat (processed)
		  Rice (processed)
		  Rye (seedless)
		  Wheat (refined)

Exclude:
  All whole nuts
  All whole seeds
	Exclude:
	  Beef
	  Fried meats or poultry
	  Skin-on Poultry
	  Tofu
		Exclude:
		  Barley
		  Oats (whole)
		  Wheat (sprouted, whole)

What are the benefits and risks of the bland diet?

The general premise of the bland diet is to provide nutrients to the person without the additional substances that can cause digestive issues. It is geared for people with digestion problems, including nausea, diarrhea, loss of appetite, or changes in taste. That is why medical providers are inclined to recommend the bland diet for those getting treatment for diseases where a side effect might be digestive distress (i.e., chemotherapy, bariatric surgery) and can be integrated into a liquid diet (see *Have a Drink*) as a way to make sure that the person will not become malnourished or suffer from wasting during treatment.

Outside of medical treatment, there are subgroups of humans that try to live anti-esthetic and anti-hedonistic lives. Where the focus is on spiritual growth independent of experiencing "joys" of life, including joys that might come from foods and from cooking. Because of the mild seasoning and limited textures of food within the bland diet, the diet has become a dogma for some who see food as a means to simply obtain nutrients and to eliminate any bliss or pleasure from food.

There are two distinct disadvantages to following a bland diet. The lack of variety in foods and flavors can make the bland diet very monotonous. Without having continuous encouragement and reinforcement to follow this diet, it can easily lead to withdrawal from the dietary practice of the bland diet. Lack of a stimulating bliss point response and triggering a reward response make it very easy to stop any new diet or optional changes to a diet and return to any other diet practice that one might be more inclined to choose. Thus, making the bland diet a very difficult diet to voluntarily follow for any long periods of time. Additionally, the low fiber content and low hydration recommendation within meals mean that someone using the bland diet can very easily become constipated. Which is why it is very important to drink fluids throughout the day as a way to ease constipation without the addition of fiber to the diet.

What does science say about the bland diet?

From the scientific evidence, there are two generalizations that can be formed about the bland diet. The use of the bland diet has been shown to be beneficial for people you suffer from digestive diseases and distress, including irritable bowel, gastric reflux and GERD, and colitis. There are also benefits from a bland diet to combat overeating and binge eating issues, when food loses its hedonistic pleasure. For those that use the bland diet to limit overeating or binge eating issues, there is an indication for reduced food consumption and it has been associated with weight loss when used in conjunction with a holistic treatment of lifestyle modification.

What can we say about the bland diet?

The bland food diet has a number of benefits for those that suffer from digestive distress or have adverse responses to spicy foods. There are also benefits that can be seen from those that exhibit binge eating and overeating issues due to the hedonistic effect that eating can have on food consumption, which may allow weight loss. Outside of these specific populations, there really is no benefit to using the bland diet or bland food diet.

Pros

- Diet is composed of foods that have high nutrient value that are easy to digest and absorb, limiting the likelihood of having nutrient deficits.
- Diet is necessary for those that experience digestive distress issues (irritable bowel, GERD) and can provide benefits to those that wish to remove the hedonistic effect from eating when attempting to lose weight.
- Diet is very economical and is generally easy to follow for anyone that wishes to use the bland diet.

Cons

- Very low palatability of the foods and low bliss response lead to a very exclusionary diet that is difficult to follow for long periods without external reinforcement and coercion
- Extremely low fiber can lead to increased risk for constipation and impaction of the colon

Blood type Diets

The premise that the blood type diet is founded on is that a person's blood type becomes the most important determinant for a healthy diet. From this single factor, proponents and apostles of the diet dogma preach that you can determine and recommend a distinct diet for the person. But actually, it is a distinct diet that is suitable for each blood type. The first recorded notion of the blood type diet was provided by author Peter D'Adamo in the book **Eat Right for Your Type** in 1996, with the premise that blood types indicate different regions of evolutionary history for humans, with type O being speculated as the most ancient blood type, and thus should be used to determine the diet that is best based on the author's speculation as to what was historically eaten during that evolutionary stage; see Table Curious2. This premise led D'Adamo to the determination that diets should be based on the ABO blood types (i.e., Type A, Type B, Type AB, Type O) and gave rise to four types of dietary groups (i.e., agrarians, nomadic, enigmas, hunters). D'Adamo then summarizes the dietary groups as follows:

- Type A: Agrarian. Optimal health from a primarily vegetarian diet.
- Type B: Nomadic. Optimal health from a primarily high dairy diet.
- Type AB: Enigmas: Must utilize a mixture of type A and B diets.
- Type O: Hunters: Optimal health from a predominantly high-protein diet, especially carnivore diet.

Unlike many of the other diets, there is not an indication about any nutrient balance. There is also no focus on Calories or Caloric balance in the blood type diet. The idea here is that health and fitness is based on the ability to match the foods and food groups that you are eating with your body's ability to process the foods at an optimal level; see Table Curious2. A relationship that is based on genetic heritage that is determined by your blood type and the idea that a molecule known as lectin will ultimately determine the health consequence of eating any specific foods from the various food groups. With the premise that lectins will interact with blood cells and trigger a cascade of physiological responses in the body leading to a host of non-commun cable diseases (i.e., cardiovascular disease, overfatness and obesity, cancer). Thereby, if someone minimes these interactions, they are able to prevent the disease from forming.

Table Curious2. Summary of primary foods that are inherently best or that should be avoided based on the person's blood type

Blood Type	Exclude	Include	
Type A	**Vegetables:** Eggplant, Legumes (Lima beans, Garbanzo beans), Tomato	**Vegetables:** Artichokes, Broccoli, Cabbage, Carrots, Celery, Fennel, Garlic, Kale, Legumes (adzuki beans, peas, black-eyed peas, soybeans) Lentils, Lettuce, Onions, Pumpkin, Spinach, Squash **Fruits:** Apricots, Blueberries, Cherries, Figs, Grapefruits, Olives, Pineapples **Nuts and Seeds (along with oil and butters):** Walnut, Flaxseed, Peanut, Pumpkin	**Grains (and flours):** Brown Rice, Buckwheat, Oat, Spelt **Meats or Alternatives:** Eggs, Fish (Cod, Salmon, Trout), Tofu, Tempeh **Dairy:** Plant-based beverages and dairy, Goat and Feta Cheese
Type B	**Vegetable:** Corn, Soy, Lentils **Meat:** Chicken	**Vegetables:** Beets, Broccoli, Cabbage, Carrots, Eggplants, Kale, Legumes (Kidney beans, Navy beans), Parsley, Peppers, Sweet Potatoes **Fruits:** Bananas, Cherries, Grapes, Olives, Pineapple, Watermelon **Nuts and Seeds (along with oil and butters):** Walnuts, Almonds, Grains (and flours): Brown rice, Oat, Millet, Spelt	**Meat or Alternative:** Eggs, Fish (Cod, Flounder, Halibut, Mahi-Mahi, Salmon, Tuna), Meat (Lamb, Venison, Turkey), **Dairy:** Animal-derived milk and yogurt, Cheese (Cottage, Feta, Goat, Mozzarella, Ricotta)

(cont)

	Avoid	Beneficial	Neutral
Type AB	**Vegetables:** Corn, Fava Bean **Fruit:** Banana **Meat:** Chicken	**Vegetables:** Beets, Broccoli, Cabbage, Carrots, Eggplants, Kale, Legumes (Kidney beans, Navy beans), Parsley, Peppers, Sweet Potatoes **Fruits:** Bananas, Cherries, Grapes, Olives, Pineapple, Watermelon	**Nuts and Seeds (along with oil and butters):** Walnuts, Almonds, Grains (and flours): Brown rice, Oat, Millet, Spelt Meat or Alternative: Eggs, Fish (Cod, Flounder, Halibut, Mahi-Mahi, Salmon, Tuna), Meat (Lamb, Venison, Turkey), **Dairy:** Animal-derived milk and yogurt, Animal-derived cheese (Cottage, Feta, Goat, Mozzarella, Ricotta)
Type O	**Vegetables:** Kidney Bean **Grains:** Wheat **Nuts and Seeds** Peanut **Oils:** Soybean oil	**Vegetables:** Artichokes, Broccoli, Kale, Legumes (adzuki beans, black-eyed peas), Lettuce, Onions, Parsley, Pumpkin, Spinach, Squash **Fruits:** Agave, Banana Blueberries, Cherries, Figs, Mangos, Olives, Watermelon	**Nuts and Seeds (along with oil and butters):** Almonds, Flaxseed, Walnut Flours: Brown Rice, Millet, Arrowroot starch **Meat (no alternatives):** Eggs, Meat (Beef, Lamb), Turkey, Fish (Cod, Halibut, Red snapper) **Dairy:** Animal-derived butter and cheese (Mozzarella, Feta)

What are the benefits of following the blood type diet?

From these interactions, the proponents of the blood type diet dogma are able to offer specific benefits to followers of the diet. There is no advertising of the diet as it relates to weight loss or weight maintenance directly, even though it is implied. With the implied reduction of lectin ingestion, there is a stipulation for a reduction in agglutination (red blood cells adhering to each other) that would keep blood flowing smoothly through the vessels and keep metabolic rates and activity at normal levels. Additionally, because of the advice to avoid processed foods and foods high in fructose combined with adherence to a regimented exercise program to increase endurance exercise, the primary benefit that proponents offer is improvement in cardiometabolic health.

What are possible risks that come from following this diet?

As with many of the dogmatic diets, there is an increased risk for nutrient deficits for those that adhere to the tenets of the blood type diet. The largest issue with deficits comes from the restriction of macronutrients that might lead to weight loss. Outside of the issue related to macronutrient deficits, the approach that people following the blood type diet makes it difficult to directly assert what deficits might arise. The increase in plant and nut consumption can lead to issues with essential fatty acid consumption and the ratio of omega-3 to omega-6, pushing us away from the 4:1 to 6:1 ratio of omega-6 to omega-3 that we strive to keep. While the proponents indicate that lectins are going to be restricted when following this diet, there are other anti-nutrients (see *Go Green...*) that can be consumed at higher rates that can disrupt digestion, absorption and availability of nutrients for the body when following the blood type diet.

What does science say about the blood type diet?

The general idea of the diet is a classical application of pseudoscience: taking some scientific idea or principle and embedding it into your argument to make the argument sound more valid. In which the tenets of the diet are based on two actual scientific ideas, genetic contribution to blood type and the presence of lectin in plants and fruits we eat. Where the premise of the diet is that blood type is determined by genetic heritage, traits, and genes passed to you through your family history is correct. But the idea that this specific genetic trait is the unique marker of evolutionary heritage that will determine metabolic health is a misguided representation of the science of genes and traits. Additionally, there are compounds referred to as lectins that are present in fruits and vegetables and can act as an anti-nutrient in our diet, a compound that interferes with digestion and absorption of nutrients, or utilization of a nutrient at a cell of the body that impacts metabolism. Yet, there is no evidence for responses to any given lectin being unique to a person's blood type or having actions that have been described by D'Adamo for reasons to follow the blood type diet. Additionally, foods listed as "best" for each blood type are known to contain high levels of lectins, even though the idea within the tenet is to avoid these foods.

With this out of the way, there is no evidence to support the claims being offered to the blood type diet. Most evidence that we have related to studies looking at the blood type diet indicates that following any of the recommendations, regardless of blood type for the person, is beneficial for the person relative to consuming foods that are processed or high in fructose. As such, the claims are not supported. Additionally, the restrictiveness of the diet can very easily lead to a number of deficiencies that are seen across the various dogmatic diets.

What can we say about the blood type diet?

There is no scientific rationale for following the blood type diet, with the major provisions of the diet paralleling many of the inclusion and exclusion of foods seen in other diets. Most of the claims of benefits come from pseudoscientific applications of human physiology and focus on personal beliefs more than any evidence that can be observed.

Pros
- Diet focuses on eating foods based on food groups and the elimination of processed and mass-produced foods that limit the consumption of metabolic disruptors that can have a positive benefit
- Unlike other diet dogmas, emphasis is placed on increasing activity and exercise as much as eating specific foods based on blood type
- Relatively easy to follow, even though highly restrictive in the recommendations, as the dietary plan is constructed with many publications being easily accessible

Cons
- There is no evidence to support the contention that blood type dictates metabolic health or metabolic effects of nutrients in the diet
- Requires taking supplements that can have adverse health effects
- Extremely restrictive, which can limit willingness to follow diet for long periods without continuous reinforcement or coercion and based on exclusion of foods among other restriction, can make the diet socially exclusionary

Gluten-Free Diets

The gluten-free diet has come to be part of a holistic treatment for people with celiac disease. Ideas that came from earlier work in the late 1880s by Samuel Gee and others that noted dietary modification with the elimination of wheat from the diet as treatment for those suffering from what we now recognize as celiac disease. Ideas resurfaced in the late 1940s and early 1950s following the publication of the work by Willem Karel Dicke, who reported that health for celiac patients improved when they avoided food that contained gluten and that was reversed when gluten was reintroduced into their daily diets.

The diet has grown as the awareness of celiac has expanded from a limited awareness to a wider acceptance of the disease. Increased awareness has been associated with an increased production of gluten-free products and a claim that following the gluten-free diet can have positive effects on overall health and be used as a successful weight loss diet without a diagnosis of celiac disease. This has led to people claiming that a gluten-free diet is important for those with non-celiac gluten sensitivity, gluten ataxia, and an allergy to wheat. The premise is that exposure to gluten will trigger an immune response within the intestines that mimics the digestive issues of those with celiac disease who are also exposed to gluten. Stemming from this claim, the tenets of the gluten-free diet have also been voluntarily adopted by a wide range of people with and without health issues; that was seen in the early 2000s with the vilification of gluten across many dietary and nutrition publications. A movement that formed the foundation for the dogma that gluten-free diets act like a "miracle drug" by those who become proponents for following a gluten-free diet. Where claims of health improvements may be related to the exclusion of processed foods that have higher amounts of gluten, but also many more metabolic disruptors that are the link with the health issues of overfatness than the "gluten-free" foods that have become ubiquitous since the early 2010s with the wider push by proponents of the diet that everyone needs to follow. A push that has led to even wider availability of gluten-free products and to eating gluten-free foods; see Table Curious3.

What are the benefits of the gluten-free diet?

To look at the claims of benefits and risks for following a gluten-free diet, it is key to understand what gluten is and why it might cause issues for people with celiac disease. Gluten is a protein that is found in barley, rye, and wheat. The gluten protein, when processed during the milling process, leads to the texture and flavor of many grain-based products (i.e., beer, breads, cakes, crackers, cookies, pizza) that we enjoy consuming. During digestion, the gluten protein will be digested similarly to other proteins, breaking the protein into its amino acids that can be absorbed without issue. But when the digestive system is overloaded with gluten, complete digestion is not achieved, and undigested gluten protein remains in the intestines. For most people, the undigested gluten protein passes easily through the intestines; yet for those with celiac disease, wheat allergies, or exhibiting gluten sensitivity the undigested gluten protein interacts with immune cells located in the intestines to cause an allergic reaction and lead to symptoms of digestive distress (i.e., irritable bowel, diarrhea, indigestion).

Table Curious3. Foods and food products that are accepted as being part of the gluten-free diet.

Foods to Avoid	Foods that might cause issues	Foods that are allowed
Grains: Barley, Durum Wheat, Einkorn Wheat, Emmer Wheat, Kamut, Oats (milled and processed), Rye, Spelt, Triticale, Wheat **Flours:** Enriched Flour, Farina, Graham Flour, Semolina **Foods and Beverages:** Beers (Ales, Lager, Porter, Stout), Breads, Cakes, Cereals, Cookies, Crackers, Croutons, Mass-produced Gravy and Sauces with Barley or Wheat binders, Malted beverages and foods, Matzo, Pasta	**Foods and Beverages:** Beers (Pilsners), Plant-based meat alternatives, Meats (Cured or Processed)	**Vegetables:** no restriction **Fruits:** no restrictions **Grains and Flours:** Amaranth, Almond Flour, Arrowroot, Buckwheat, Cornmeal/Hominy, Flaxseed, Millet, Oats (non-milled), Potato Flour, Quinoa, Rice and Rice Flour, Sorghum, Tapioca **Nuts and Seeds:** no restriction **Meats and Meat-Alternative:** Eggs, Non-processed meats, Fish (non-breaded), Poultry (non-breaded), Tofu **Dairy:** Animal-derived milk , Animal-derived dairy products, Plant-based beverages (non-malted)

The gluten-free diet will thus prevent the onset of the symptoms of digestive distress. But this would only be for those with celiac disease and would have adverse responses to the incomplete digestion of the gluten protein. Something that between 1% and 2% of all people suffer from, not nearly a large enough population to support a dogmatic diet that has within its allowed foods, to explain the cluster of mass-produced foods that net companies over $15 billion each year. So, what benefits might be available to anyone that would follow this diet?

Let's start with people that might have digestive issues similar to those suffering from celiac disease. For those that stipulate having gluten sensitivity (more on that to come), following a gluten-free diet for short periods of time can lead to improvements in digestive functions. While for those that have allergies to barley, rye, or wheat, the use of the gluten-free diet alleviates many digestive distress symptoms that accompany eating many processed foods.

Outside of the health issues related to digestive distress, what else might be a benefit to following the gluten-free diet? Similar to other dogmatic diets that limit ultra-processed foods there are metabolic and cardiometabolic changes that limit the degree of overfatness expressed by the person. These changes are seen with improved glucose metabolism and increased break down and utilization of fat for fuel. From these metabolic changes, following a gluten-free diet may result in weight loss and/or reduced body fat. The combination of reduced fat mass, normalization of adipokines (fat-cell-produced hormones), and limited ingestion of metabolic disruptors leads to reduced inflammation and improved cardiovascular health. When combined with exercise and increased physical activity, there are improvements in overall health, and, for those with athletic endeavors, there are noted improvements in athletic performance.

What about costs and risks?

These benefits do not come without costs and risks for the followers. The largest of which can be seen in the actual monetary cost for following the diet. Even though the gluten-free products have become more widely available, their share of total products is still limited, and the cost of making the products is typically higher relative to conventional products, combine to make the diet more expensive, and for those on limited income, it may not be a sustainable diet to follow. Along with all of the other dogmatic diets, there is a risk for nutrient deficiency. Based on the foods that are forbidden, those who follow gluten-free diets are at risk of not reaching recommended dietary intake for various B vitamins (e.g., B_1, B_2, B_3, B_9), coenzymes, and provitamin compounds (i.e., carotenes, flavonoids), along with several electrolytes (i.e., calcium, iron). Deficiencies that increase the risk for anemia, fatigue, increased irritability and mood swings, pellagra, reduced mental awareness and alertness, and muscle cramping.

While deficiencies can arise, the inclusion and exclusion of specific foods can lead to issues of overconsumption. The exclusion of many foods that have added fiber in them may reduce fiber and increase glycemic load with each meal. The diet also has the chance to increase the consumption of foods with higher fat content that can impact fat and cholesterol metabolism following each meal. The changes in glycemic load and fat content have the potential to lead to issues of metabolic syndrome (i.e., high blood glucose, high LDL and total cholesterol levels, and high triglyceride levels) if the diet is not balanced and regulated correctly. Additionally, with the growth of popularity and mass-produced foods for the gluten-free diet, the risk of consuming foods with metabolic disruptors increases, which can offset any potential benefit that might come from following the gluten-free diet.

Like other highly specific diets, there is the issue of social exclusion and difficulty in finding food and building meals outside of the home or very selective restaurants. This social exclusion and difficulty with finding foods make the diet very difficult to follow without continuous reinforcement and rewards to make it a self-monitored and self-selected diet.

What does science say about the gluten-free diet?

One of the major issues with the gluten-free diets is the vilification of gluten that has become the hallmark of many talking points surrounding "good" and "bad" foods that we have access to in our diet. The premise of the vilification is based on the premise that people are walking around sensitive to gluten without knowing that they are sensitive to gluten. Unfortunately, there is no evidence to support the notion that there is widespread sensitivity to gluten in humans. Additionally, many common foods seen throughout human history contain gluten and outside the recent speculation coming from the acolytes of the gluten-free diet, there is no historical evidence to support the connotation that gluten sensitivity is common, either. As such, we should be very skeptical of the claims surrounding gluten sensitivity being common and may represent a Hawthorne effect (thinking that one has something leads to seeing evidence of that thing or changes in physiology to match expected responses from that issue) at play more than actual physiological issues. There are also some proponents of the gluten-free diet that rely on the relationship reported, via correlative studies, in some very questionable studies that there is a relationship between neurological disorders (i.e., autism, schizophrenia) and a diet that includes food containing gluten. There is, however, no direct evidence to support the claims of gluten with neurological disorders based on a cause-and-effect relationship.

Additionally, there appears to a positive effect of gluten-free diets have on overfatness and other non-communicable diseases that are directly related to the reduction in foods with metabolic disruptors, and for those with high fatness and inflammation, a change in hormone signals leads to normalization of inflammation and the improvement in overall health. A lot of proponents like to link this with the diet itself, but it appears to parallel responses seen from other dogmatic diets that limit consumption of trans fats, fructose, and other metabolic disruptors rather than due to the specific tenets of the gluten-free diet.

What can we say about gluten-free diets?

The gluten-free diet has become one of the trendier diets in popular culture, with more people self-selecting to restrict gluten from their diet. However, outside of individuals with specific medical needs, there is limited evidence to support many of the claims that have made the diet so trendy.

Pros

- Relatively flexible diet with a wide array of choices for foods that can be safely followed with appropriate planning and is able to be adjusted to other dietary restrictions or nutritional treatment plans
- Diet is essential for those with celiac disease and can have benefits for those with wheat allergies or express gluten sensitivity
- Due to comorbidity between autoimmune diseases (e.g., celiac disease, type-1 diabetes, lupus, rheumatoid arthritis), the use of gluten-free diets may be beneficial in the nutritional treatment of other diseases
- Associated with improved athletic performance when combined with an appropriate training regimen and volumes

Cons

- Diet can lead to nutrient deficits and diseases of nutrient deficiencies, but at the same time, it without proper planning may contain foods high in fat and fruits that have a glycemic index and tend to be low in fiber that increase the risk for developing metabolic issues if followed for very-long periods.
- Even though trendy, the diet can be socially exclusionary as the choices being offered at restaurants are limited and gluten-free foods have lower bliss response and subsequent appeal for consuming.
- Because of the trendiness and the increased availability of mass-produced and processed gluten-free foods, the consumption of metabolic disruptors can increase, which lead to the development of health issues associated with overfatness.

Take-home message

What can be said about our curious dogmatic diets? Outside of suffering from specific digestive diseases, there really is no scientifically valid reason for following the dogmatic tenets of either the bland food or gluten-free diets. While there really is not a lot of harm that can come from following these diets and we have a lot of anecdotes and correlative benefits to following the diets, unless you would self-select for following these two diets, it is not a diet that should be dogmatically followed to every tenet. At the same time, should you self-select to follow these diets without medical necessity, it is important to plan the diet correctly to minimize any adverse effects of development of nutrient deficiencies that can arise from either diet.

As for the blood type diet, well, let's just follow the advice of Nancy Reagan and "just say no." There is no rationale to follow the blood type diet. The central tenets advocated are based on personal beliefs that are not supported in any way and can lead to an excessively restrictive diet that can do more harm than good.

A final take home message.

*"Preach not to others what they should eat, but eat
as becomes you, and be silent."*
—Epicurus, 55-135 C.E. date of quote not cited.

Given all of the various dogmatic perspectives and tenets to follow, there is one last question to answer... *is there really a best diet, a best dogma, to believe in?*

If we are to follow the trend that has been seen throughout the book, and with most things dealing with how the body works. The answer is **it depends**. Because the response here is that it depends, we get trapped into what we want to believe is best about our dogma versus some other dogma, based on what we want to believe is the best.

So, instead of answering that there is or is not a best diet, I want to address a point that I have been thinking about for a few years now. That maybe we need to start thinking differently about the way we go about dieting that could be better than, say, one dogma versus another. In my argument here, I will be focused on a concept that has come to the forefront of my idea about getting the most appropriate response for exercise. If we want to consistently see improvements, then we need to incorporate periodization into the program. Periodization allows for changing the stress of exercise so that the body is constantly attempting to adapt to new demands, and stagnation is not possible.

An idea not presented when discussing the idea of diets or dieting, leading to my favorite question... ***but* why?**

Why is periodization of diets not as regularly recommended to the same extent that periodization of exercise gets recommended?

A lot of the answer lies in the perception that we have about diet and the idea that consistency in diet is important in establishing optimal performance and essential for good health. Ideals that focused on discussions about diets as needing to be individually tailored to meet specific metabolic demands. Even so, these ideals of individually tailoring diets tend to not look at metabolic demands but instead to follow established guidelines for consuming macronutrients (carbohydrates, proteins, and lipids), vitamins, and minerals that are not based on metabolic demand but on the amount needed relative to body mass or by a percentage of total Caloric intake for a day.

My recommendation here will try to present an ideal that does not overtly emphasize dietary stipulations and recommendations may fall along the lines of needing to follow specific dietary patterns to meet some sort of cultural standard. As cultural standards have importance in each of our lives, they should always be integrated into whatever we are doing with our friends and family. And more importantly, I am going to make every attempt possible to ignore the dietary ideals and tenets that align with what is deemed as being socially correct for a type of person based on weight, gender, or body image, or agree with the ever-present dietary trends pitched by our favorite self-appointed influencers of social media feeds. Such actions have the potential to propagate fad diets or may instill cognitive drivers and reinforcers known to elicit body image (body dysmorphic) issues and eating patterns that mimic having anorexia or bulimia.

The idea here is to actually focus on the idea of diet in the context of our long-term goals, and then it would make sense to alter the diet sporadically to meet the changes in our metabolic demands. Or possibly force a change in our metabolic demands based on changes in nutrient load from our diet. Where we have to recall that availability of nutrients directly impacts metabolism and performance by influencing muscle strength, muscle endurance, metabolic flexibility, cardiovascular/aerobic endurance, immune response to stress, and neurological (cognitive) function.

As such, I would like to recommend a different approach. A periodized approach to diet that utilizes an approach to diet that would allow for variability in nutrients based on addressing the following core ideas to determine proportions and ratios within any meal based on the following factors:

- o What is my nutrient balance point based on my metabolic demands? See the appendix for noted balance points for micronutrients base on age and socially identified genders
- o How many meals will I have throughout the day?
- o What is the quality of the nutrients in the foods that I am choosing to eat?

And not focus on key tenets or core dogmatic principles that need to be followed in order to "correctly" use any of the diets that we commonly are thinking about trying or are currently following.

Even though these questions have been addressed in earlier points throughout this book (along with my musing on the podcast and YouTube videos), the idea of manipulating our responses to the questions based on the concepts of periodization has not been addressed. What is interesting is that this idea is not regularly found anywhere in the research literature, so I am going to get a little speculative here and answer the question. What might happen by following a periodized approach to diet in the same way that we might for exercise?

While there are speculations stemming from research about the use of periodization of diet for athletic performance, there is little in this regard for everyone else. Athletic performance improves when diet is modified to meet the specific demands of the period of training (i.e., hypertrophy or growth, increased strength, improved endurance, aesthetic changes). But what if we are not athletes? To extrapolate from the information available, the easy answer is that we should be able to get through points of stagnation in our improvements in health or weight loss or limit negative reinforcers that restrictive diets might impart. Changes are needed, as we know that most diets "fail" in the long term because of the restrictiveness that diets place on the person's overall lifestyle or the sense of coercion that is imparted on the dieter in order to continue the diet, which makes it less likely to be used without supervision. Thus, making changes in diet can encourage continuous adaptations (i.e., muscle growth, weight loss, body compositional changes) and improvements in performance (i.e., gains in strength, endurance, or power).

Can we develop a periodized diet?

To start, let's reflect on four patterns for periodized diets that we have research on. All four predominantly reflect the consumption of sugar in the diet or the faulty evaluation of caloric intake and are described as "train high, compete high" where the diet is a high-carbohydrate diet with additional carbohydrate intake before, during, and after training that is meant to ensure glycogen content remains high, "train low, compete high" where the diet is a low-carbohydrate diet for 7 to 10 days of training that is followed by three days of "carbo-loading" using a high-carbohydrate diet and is meant to replenish and grow glycogen stores, "recover low, sleep low" where a low-carbohydrate diet is followed during the afternoon or evening and is meant to deplete glycogen stores and when carbohydrates become available lead to greater glycogen storage, or "sleep low, train low" where carbohydrate intake is restricted in the afternoon and night to deplete muscle glycogen leading to mourning exercise session that is followed by consuming carbohydrate intake after the training session and is meant to replenish and grow glycogen stores. The idea presented in each of the four diets is that altering metabolism for a very short period of time leads to an increased fat utilization and transition into a ketogenic state.

Most of this research has been on athletic endeavors and improving endurance performance and has not direct evidence for the ability to change body mass or body composition. Yet, the world of bodybuilding has used some of the principles of the research and integrated them into long-standing practices of bulks and cuts. Periods of gaining weight, where consumption of all macronutrients is in excess of balance points, are followed by periods of extreme restrictions to macronutrients, especially carbohydrates, where a diet mimics a "carnivore" diet, with the intention to not cause weight loss but instead a reduction in fat mass. These ideas have become more mainstream with the integration of the training concepts related to bodybuilding becoming the primary application of exercise prescription in gymnasiums and fitness centers, or from the social media feeds of many self-reported experts of fitness. This idea of bulks and cuts for bodybuilders takes a third stage mimicking the carbo-loading diet of endurance athletes for the 10 days leading into competition. Where for seven days one follows a low-carbohydrate diet while training at high intensities, it is then followed by 3 days of low-intensity training and eating a high-carbohydrate or a high-starch diet leading into showcases and performance. This phase of the bodybuilding periodization is meant to increase the glycogen stores and water within the skeletal muscles to enhance overall physique and is generally not followed when we look at periodization of diets outside of athletes or bodybuilders.

What can be said about the notion to periodize diets?

So, to the question of can we periodize the diet? The answer is a resounding yes! But that just leads to the next question…

How to periodize the diet?

We can integrate periodization into our diet without focusing on the restriction of calories or carbohydrates, and just like with our exercise periodization, it all starts with goal development and timelines. Falling back on what was shown for when we should see responses and when responses will reach their peak and plateau, meaning we need to break our calendars into 4-week and then into 8-to-12-week windows. Where noticeable responses will be seen by 4 weeks and plateaus will be reached between week 8 and week 12, and thus changes in diet should correspond to these time frames.

For those who have found a diet that they prefer to follow, integrating short-term (i.e., 1- or 2-week) "cutting" patterns into their diet before returning to their preferred diet can be beneficial. One such change can be the brief use of alternate-day fasting or time-restricted feeding, changes that have been indicated to have the benefits of improving one's metabolic health with a side effect of aesthetic changes (i.e., reduction of fat mass). Another possible means to integrate periodization into diet is to incorporate a ketogenic approach, where (using Atkins-style terminology) you integrate an introduction phase of 3 days of excessively low carbohydrates (i.e., 10-15 grams per day) followed by slowly re-instituting carbohydrates at growing levels of 20-100 grams per day over the next week, which can lead to changes in metabolic functions and increase fat utilization and a reduction of fat mass. Eventually leading up to consuming at least minimal levels of carbohydrates (120-130 grams per day) needed for proper metabolic functions and optimal performance of our nervous system.

It is important that during these changes, your exercise program changes to help maximize the metabolic responses that you are causing. While at the same time, coming out of these brief changes in diet, you are not overconsuming food to offset the lack of nutrition during the "cut" phases.

On the other hand, instead of following a "cut" phase mentality, we can incorporate an ever-evolving dietary pattern. A pattern that uses an 8-12 week timeframe to change dietary principles where we go through different diets (e.g., intermittent fasting or time-restricted feeding to ketogenic to proportional diet to vegetarian) in an order where at the end of each window and during our training transitions we use a "free eating" where there are no restrictions (outside of ensuring minimal and maximal are taken into consideration) on what type of food is being eaten or when meals take place, followed by the next dietary period. A pattern of dietary and exercise modifications that should help to provide the necessary physiological stimulus for continuous changes to be seen (or at least minimize the effects of plateauing) along with providing a cognitive reinforcer for continuing dieting in the long term, far after the sense of restrictiveness or social exclusion might have triggered our stopping.

What must be stipulated here is that the restrictions and changes in diet need to be reflective of the appropriate cognitive drive. A cognitive drive that does not focus on comparison of body image to someone else, focus on the weight reading displayed on a scale, or attempt to equate Calories between what is being consumed with what is being expended in exercise. Keeping this stipulation in mind is important, as we want to make these changes without causing the sensation of body dysmorphia to take hold or instigating an exercise bulimic response.

We know that periodization works. It works in our exercise regimen to make sure that we are not overtraining and that we can see consistent gains towards our overall goals. There is some evidence to support the use of periodization for our diets too if we can follow a planned strategy to modify our diets either in response to each period of our training regimen or based on the principles of when we see responses and when responses will plateau.

Integrating a periodized approach can not only help with enhancing adaptations from exercise but can also help with overcoming the cognitive desire to stop dieting or exercising prior to reaching our long-term goals. This periodization can be as simple as integrating breaks into our regular dietary plan by introducing "cut" phases through either intermittent fasting or short-term ketogenic dietary patterns, or as complex as establishing a rotating dietary pattern with "free eating" weeks that correspond with the transition periods between our moderate-term goals. The whole idea here is to approach diet in the same manner as we approach exercise, where if we want to achieve our long-term goals, it means incorporating self-selected dietary patterns that offer breaks from the feelings of restrictiveness, whether they are sensed socially, cognitively, or physiologically.

One final-take home message... a closing argument, if you will, about the dogmatic diets

Well, here we are... the end of the story about dogmatic diets? Throughout the discussion, we continually looked at dogmatic tenets that are embedded into the various diets with the implicit intention to make it feel like it's "us" versus "them" when it comes time to choose the appropriate diet to believe in and follow. An implicit intention that has been used throughout human history to generate culture and, from culture, religion. I intentionally skimmed through the impact of religion in making dogmatic diets, even though we do have evidence to show that, like other diets, following some of the religious diets can influence how we talk about food, lead to nutrient deficits, and may impact our health just like all of the other diets. Yet, we must also note that embedding one's religious practices and tenets into selecting food can also lead to the selection of food that will minimize exposure to foods containing metabolic disruptors and might have some health benefits.

But we might want to step back and revisit the opening question. Are diets our new religion?

The answer is … yes … no … well, maybe. It really depends on how we want to talk about diets and the perspective that we have about our food and how we eat. Perspectives that can also be seen within religious practices regarding inclusion and exclusion of foods, food groups, food preparation, and meal planning. Perspectives about diets and dietary practices have been used throughout time, mostly because religions and diets have evolved with each other and formed the way we tend to talk about our food. Religious approaches that have been co-opted into the way that fad diets approach building their messaging as a way to build a community and instill the psychological benefits of belonging. Where, yes, some diets that will incorporate the 3 aspects of religion, dietary practices such as veganism when followed orthodoxically, go beyond diet itself and incorporate the primary tenets into every aspect of life and lifestyle that it takes the shape of culture and from a pseudo-religion. A perspective that sometimes is the fundamental rationale for avoiding discussing anything about veganism out of fear of being preached to by those that follow the vegan lifestyle.

Yet, even if fad diets are not religions, they add something that many religions have done throughout history. They have added their cultural overtones to society and impact how we talk about diets, nutrition, and even metabolism. They not only change how we talk about foods but also instill a sense of morality to the foods that we eat. In some sense, we use fad diet dogmas to give us a sense of guilt or feelings of superiority, based solely on our food choices. This sense of well-being comes with words and ideas that have only recently been coined to explain the dogmas of the fad diets. Words and ideas that most likely would not be readily recognizable if not for the catalog of fad diets that we get exposed to on a daily basis.

Would we even have seen the debates in December, 2023 about the value of whole milk versus fat-free milk in the halls of the United States Congress if it were not for the low-fat dietary dogmas influencing public policy? Would we see public comments surrounding the assumption that the same foods are automatically unhealthy when cooked at a fast-food restaurant while they somehow become healthy when cooked at home, the hysteria about GMO foods, or the hypervigilance that some parents have about sugar in anything a kid eats, if it were not for the low-fat, low-sugar, all-natural/organic fad diet proponents and zealots? I mean, heck, I've even seen products like table salt and bottled-water being labeled on the shelves of a grocery store as "natural" and "gluten-free" simply to appease the followers of those dietary dogmas.

Which leads me to my closing statement. **Follow the diet you like, but don't preach at your friends, family, colleagues, or if you're an educator, to your students about what diet they should follow.** We need to relax a little and stop with the zealotry about diets and approach this idea with an open-minded. The zealotry and egotism of needing to be right about diets have led us to doing some really idiotic things when it comes to our food and how we interact with others when it comes to our food choices. Everything here is about choices, and every diet that we try to dogmatically follow has both pros and cons, so when you make your choices, make the best choice... remembering that there are no "good" foods or "bad" foods, there is only food if we try to avoid being dogmatic.

Yes, there are medical reasons for needing to use a specific diet or avoid a specific food... but unless you are one of the individuals that actually suffer from those afflictions, there really isn't a reason to be a zealot for the diet. But more importantly, to be a zealot against someone else's diet... severe food allergies are life-threatening issues, and we should be a little more compassionate and empathetic to these people.

We have to remember that there will always be a "new" fad diets. New fads, like most of the fads we are seeing today, will most likely be just simply rebrands of older fads. Because we live within a society that may not have been taught anything about the history of lifestyle trends, or that does not remember having seen the older fads.

And finally, this time I mean it: while there could be some benefits from using the principles of the fad diet, if claims being offered sound extraordinary, then we should expect to see extraordinary evidence from research leading to a consensus that yes, you will see extraordinary results. And speaking of results, it is especially important to realize that everyone will respond in some way along a continuum of possible responses to every dietary intervention; it is all a matter of how much response occurs or how much time it takes to when each of us will see results...

Acknowledgements

As with everything I do, this could not have been completed without assistance. I need to first thank all of my former students that have put up with me going on random tangents related to diet, nutrition and metabolism, that challenged and debated me on the points about their specific diets and lifestyles that have been covered in this book. Without their intellectual curiosities I don't think I would have taken time to put my ideas formerly down and eventually type them into the book that you have read.

I would be remised to not directly thank people who have taken time out of their lives to read through the discussions and help me out, making sure that thoughts are clear and understandable, especially Ashley Viveros, Britney Mendoza, Martha Wiszniak, and Makayla Sousa. I also need to direct a big thanks to Ricci Bicomong, Ashley Viveros, Makayla Sousa, and Dalton Joliette who were each kind enough to join me in recording several episodes of the podcast that became part of the book.

Appendix A:

Generalized micronutrient (mineral/electrolyte) balance points (grams/day) based on recognized adequate intake values for age range and social gender identifications. (Source: National Institutes of Health, Office of Dietary Supplements https://ods.od.nih.gov/HealthInformation/nutrientrecommendations.aspx)

Age and Gender	Calcium (mg/d)	Chromium (µg/d)	Copper (µg/d)	Fluoride (mg/d)	Iodine (µg/d)	Iron (mg/d)	Magnesium (mg/d)	Manganese (mg/d)	Molybdenum (µg/d)	Phosphorus (mg/d)	Selenium (µg/d)	Zinc (mg/d)	Potassium (mg/d)	Sodium (mg/d)	Chloride (g/d)
0–6 mo.	200	0.2	200	0.01	110	0.27	30	0.003	2	100	15	2	400	110	0.18
7–12 mo.	260	5.5	220	0.5	130	11	75	0.6	3	275	20	3	860	370	0.57
1–3 yr	700	11	340	0.7	90	7	80	1.2	17	460	20	3	2,000	800	1.5
4–8 yr	1,000	15	440	1	90	10	130	1.5	22	500	30	5	2,300	1,000	1.9
9–13 yr															
Males	1,300	25	700	2	120	8	240	1.9	34	1,250	40	8	2,500	1,200	2.3
Females	1,300	21	700	2	120	8	240	1.6	34	1,250	40	8	2,300	1,200	2.3
14–18 y															
Males	1,300	35	890	3	150	11	410	2.2	43	1,250	55	11	3,000	1,500	2.3
Females	1,300	24	890	3	150	15	360	1.6	43	1,250	55	9	2,300	1,500	2.3
19–30 y															
Males	1,000	35	900	4	150	8	400	2.3	45	700	55	11	3,400	1,500	2.3
Females	1,000	25	900	3	150	18	310	1.8	45	700	55	8	2,600	1,500	2.3
31–50 y															
Males	1,000	35	900	4	150	8	420	2.3	45	700	55	11	3,400	1,500	2.3
Females	1,000	25	900	3	150	18	320	1.8	45	700	55	8	2,600	1,500	2.3
51–70 y															
Males	1,000	30	900	4	150	8	420	2.3	45	700	55	11	3,400	1,500	2
Females	1,200	20	900	3	150	8	320	1.8	45	700	55	8	2,600	1,500	2
> 70 y															
Males	1,200	30	900	4	150	8	420	2.3	45	700	55	11	3,400	1,500	1.8
Females	1,200	20	900	3	150	8	320	1.8	45	700	55	8	2,600	1,500	1.8

Appendix B:

Generalized micronutrient (vitamin) balance points (grams/day) based on the recognized adequate intake values for age range and social gender identifications. (Source: National Institutes of Health, Office of Dietary Supplements

Age and Gender	Vitamin A (µg/d)	Vitamin C (mg/d)	Vitamin D (µg/d)	Vitamin E (mg/d)	Vitamin K (µg/d)	Vitamin B1 (mg/d)	Vitamin B2 (mg/d)	Vitamin B3 (mg/d)	Vitamin B5 (mg/d)	Vitamin B6 (mg/d)	Vitamin B7 (µg/d)	Vitamin B9 (µg/d)	Vitamin B12 (µg/d)	Choline (mg/d)
0–6 mo	400	40	10	4	2.0	0.2	0.3	2	1.7	0.1	5	65	0.4	125
6–12 mo	500	50	10	5	2.5	0.3	0.4	4	1.8	0.3	6	80	0.5	150
1–3 yr	300	15	15	6	30	0.5	0.5	6	2	0.5	8	150	0.9	200
4–8 yr	400	25	15	7	55	0.6	0.6	8	3	0.6	12	200	1.2	250
9–13 yr														
Males	600	45	15	11	60	0.9	0.9	12	4	1.0	20	300	1.8	375
Females	600	45	15	11	60	0.9	0.9	12	4	1.0	20	300	1.8	375
14–18 yr														
Males	900	75	15	15	75	1.2	1.3	16	5	1.3	25	400	2.4	550
Females	700	65	15	15	75	1.0	1.0	14	5	1.2	25	400	2.4	400
19–30 yr														
Males	900	90	15	15	120	1.2	1.3	16	5	1.3	30	400	2.4	550
Females	700	75	15	15	90	1.1	1.1	14	5	1.3	30	400	2.4	425
31–50 yr														
Males	900	90	15	15	120	1.2	1.3	16	5	1.3	30	400	2.4	550
Females	700	75	15	15	90	1.1	1.1	14	5	1.3	30	400	2.4	425
51–70 yr														
Males	900	90	15	15	120	1.2	1.3	16	5	1.7	30	400	2.4	550
Females	700	75	15	15	90	1.1	1.1	14	5	1.5	30	400	2.4	425
> 70 yr														
Males	900	90	20	15	120	1.2	1.3	16	5	1.7	30	400	2.4	550
Females	700	75	20	15	90	1.1	1.1	14	5	1.5	30	400	2.4	425

Appendix C:

Changes in generalized micronutrient balance points (grams/day) based on the recognized adequate intake values for pregnancy or during lactation and breastfeeding. (Source: National Institutes of Health, Office of Dietary Supplements https://ods.od.nih.gov/HealthInformation/nutrientrecommendations.aspx)

Age	Vitamin A (µg/d)	Vitamin C (mg/d)	Vitamin D (µg/d)	Vitamin E (mg/d)	Vitamin K (µg/d)	Vitamin B1 (mg/d)	Vitamin B2 (mg/d)	Vitamin B3 (mg/d)	Vitamin B5 (mg/d)	Vitamin B6 (mg/d)	Vitamin B7 (µg/d)	Vitamin B9 (µg/d)	Vitamin B12 (µg/d)	Choline (mg/d)
14–18 yr														
Pregnancy	750	80	15	15	75	1.4	1.4	18	6	1.9	30	600	2.6	450
Lactation	1,200	115	15	19	75	1.4	1.6	17	7	2.0	35	500	2.8	550
19–30 yr														
Pregnancy	770	85	15	15	90	1.4	1.4	18	6	1.9	30	600	2.6	450
Lactation	1,300	120	15	19	90	1.4	1.6	17	7	2.0	35	500	2.8	550
31–50 yr														
Pregnancy	770	85	15	15	90	1.4	1.4	18	6	1.9	30	600	2.6	450
Lactation	1,300	120	15	19	90	1.4	1.6	17	7	2.0	35	500	2.8	550

Age	Calcium (mg/d)	Chromium (µg/d)	Copper (µg/d)	Fluoride (mg/d)	Iodine (µg/d)	Iron (mg/d)	Magnesium (mg/d)	Manganese (mg/d)	Molybdenum (µg/d)	Phosphorus (mg/d)	Selenium (µg/d)	Zinc (mg/d)	Potassium (mg/d)	Sodium (mg/d)	Chloride (g/d)
14–18 y															
Pregnancy	1,300	29	1,000	3	220	27	400	2.0	50	1,250	60	12	2,600	1,500	2.3
Lactation	1,300	44	1,300	3	290	10	360	2.6	50	1,250	70	13	2,500	1,500	2.3
19–30 y															
Pregnancy	1,000	30	1,000	3	220	27	350	2.0	50	700	60	11	2,900	1,500	2.3
Lactation	1,000	45	1,300	3	290	9	310	2.6	50	700	70	12	2,800	1,500	2.3
31–50 y															
Pregnancy	1,000	30	1,000	3	220	27	360	2.0	50	700	60	11	2,900	1,500	2.3
Lactation	1,000	45	1,300	3	290	9	320	2.6	50	700	70	12	2,800	1,500	2.3

References

Diets, it's our new religion

1. Abdollahpouri H, Burke R, Mansoury M, Mobasher B. The unfairness of popularity bias in recommendation. 2019;13th ACM Conference on Recommender Systems. Copenhagen, Denmark.
2. Beaulieu DA, Best LA. Eat, pray, love: disordered eating in religious and non-religious men and women. J Eat Disord. 2022;10, 198. DOI:10.1186/s40337-022-00721-8
3. Chouraqui JP, Turck D, Briend A, et al. Religious dietary rules and their potential nutritional and health consequences. Int J Epidemiol. 2021;50(1):12-26. DOI:10.1093/ije/dyaa182.
4. Cohen AB. You can learn a lot about religion from food. Current Opinion in Psychology. 2021;40, 1-5. DOI:10.1016/j.copsyc.2020.07.032
5. Frankle RT, Heussenstamm FK. Food zealotry and youth: new dilemmas for professionals. Am J Public Health. 1974;64(1):11-8. DOI:10.2105/ajph.64.1.1
6. Jovanovski N, Jaeger T. Demystifying 'diet culture': Exploring the meaning of diet culture in online 'anti-diet' feminist, fat activist, and health professional communities. Women's Studies International Forum. 2022; 90. DOI: 10.1016/j.wsif.2021.102558.
7. Lelwica M. The religion of thinness. *Scripta Instituti Donneriani Aboensis. 2011;23*, 257–285. DOI:10.30674/scripta.67400
8. Raiter N, Husundinov R, Mazza K, Lamarcher L. TikTok promotes diet culture and negative body image rhetoric: A content analysis. Journal of Nutrition Education and Behavior. 2023; 55(10), 755-760. DOI: 10.1016/j.neb.2023.08.001
9. Thircuir S. I eat therefore I believe: The raw food diet, a believing solution for healing. The International Journal of Religion and Spirituality in Society. 2019;9(1), 41-55. DOI:10.18848/21548633/CGP/v09i01/41-55
10. Zeller B. Totem and taboo in the grocery store: quasi-religious foodways in North America. *Scripta Instituti Donneriani Aboensis.* 2015;*26*, 11–31. DOI:10.30674/scripta.67444

Calories go in ... Calories go out...

1. Aragon, A.A., et al., *International society of sports nutrition position stand: diets and body composition.* Journal of the International Society of Sports Nutrition, 2022. **14**(1)
2. American College of Sports Medicine, American Dietetic Association, Dieticians of Canda. Nutrition and Athletic Performance. Med. Sci. Sports Exerc. Feb 6 2009.
3. American Dietetic Association. Position of the American Dietetic Association: Health Implications of Dietary Fiber. J. Am. Diet. Assoc. 2008;108(10):1716-1731.
4. American Dietetic Association. Position of the American Dietetic Association: Nutrient Supplementation. J. Am. Diet. Assoc. 2009;109(12):2073-2085.
5. American Dietetic Association, Dieticians of Canda, American College of Sports Medicine. Position of the American Dietetic Association, Dietitians of Canada, and the American College of Sports Medicine: Nutrition and Athletic Performance. J. Am. Diet. Assoc. 2009;109(3):509-527.
6. American Dietetic Association and American Society for Nutrition. Position of the American Dietetic Association and American Society for Nutrition: Obesity, Reproduction, and Pregnancy Outcomes. J. Am. Diet. Assoc. 2009;109(5):918-927.
7. American Heart Association Nutrition Committee, Lichtenstein AH, Appel LJ, et al. Diet and lifestyle recommendations revision 2006: a scientific statement from the American Heart Association Nutrition Committee. Circulation. Jul 4 2006;114(1):82-96
8. Brown RE, Canning KL, Fung M, et al. Calorie Estimation in Adults Differing in Body Weight Class and Weight Loss Status. *Med Sci Sports Exerc.* Mar 2016;48(3):521-526.
9. Burke LM, Winter JA, Cameron-Smith D, Enslen M, Farnfield MM, Decombaz J. Effect of intake of different dietary protein sources on plasma amino acid profiles at rest and after exercise. Int. J. Sport Nutr. Exerc. Metab. 2012;22(6):452-462.
10. Campbell B, Kreider RB, Ziegenfuss TN, et al. International Society of Sports Nutrition position stand: protein and exercise. J. Int. Soc. Sports Nutr. 2007;4(8).
11. Carbone JW, Pasiakos SM. Dietary Protein and Muscle Mass: Translating Science to Application and Health Benefit. Nutrients. May 22 2019;11(5).
12. Cheuvront SN. The Zone Diet phenomenon: a closer look at the science behind the claims. J. Am. Coll. Nutr. Feb 1 2003;22(1):9-17.
13. Ciuris C, Lynch HM, Wharton C, Johnston CS. A Comparison of Dietary Protein Digestibility, Based on DIAAS Scoring, in Vegetarian and Non-Vegetarian Athletes. Nutrients. Dec 10 2019;11(12).
14. Clark JE. An overview of the contribution of fatness and fitness factors, and the role of exercise, in the formation of health status for individuals who are overweight. J. Diabetes Metab. Disord. Jan 1 2012;11(1):19.
15. Clark JE. Metabolism and nutrition: integration of concepts in a holistic approach to teaching metabolism. HAPS Educator. 2021;25(2):82-102.
16. Clark JE. Diets and Diet Therapy: Diet Supplements for Exercise. In: Ferranti P, Berry EM, Anderson JR, eds. Encyclopedia of Food Security and Sustainability. Vol 2: Elsevier; 2019:161-170.
17. Clark JE, Sirois E. Coercion versus self-selection when treating issues of overfatness: A narrative review. Health Educ. J. 2023:1-12.
18. Coyle EF, Jeukendrup AE, Oseto MC, Hodgkinson BJ, Zderic TW. Low-fat diet alters intramuscular substrates and reduces lipolysis and fat oxidation during exercise. Am. J. Physiol. Endocrinol. Metab. Mar 1 2001;280(3):E391-398.

19. Curi R, Newsholme P, Marzuca-Nassr GN, et al. Regulatory principles in metabolism-then and now. Biochem. J. Jul 1 2016;473(13):1845-1857.

20. Da Poian AT, El-Bacha T, Luz MRMP. Nutrient utilization in humans: metabolism pathways. Nature Education. 2010;3(9):11.

21. Fern EB, Watzke H, Barclay DV, Roulin A, Drewnowski A. The Nutrient Balance Concept: A New Quality Metric for Composite Meals and Diets. PLoS One. 2015;10(7):e0130491.

22. Freeland-Graves JH, Nitzke S, Academy of N, Dietetics. Position of the academy of nutrition and dietetics: total diet approach to healthy eating. J. Acad. Nutr. Diet. Feb 2013;113(2):307-317.

23. Fuchs CJ, Gonzalez JT, van Loon LJC. Fructose co-ingestion to increase carbohydrate availability in athletes. J. Physiol. Jul 2019;597(14):3549-3560.

24. Hall KD. What is the required energy deficit per unit weight loss? Int. J. Obes. (Lond.). Mar 2008;32(3):573-576.

25. Hawley JA, Hargreaves M, Zierath JR. Signalling mechanisms in skeletal muscle: role in substrate selection and muscle adaptation. Essays Biochem. 2006;42:1-12.

26. Henry CJK. Basal metabolic rate studies in humans: measurement and development of new equations Public Health Nutr. 2007;8(7a):1133-1152.

27. Herman MA, Samuel VT. The Sweet Path to Metabolic Demise: Fructose and Lipid Synthesis. Trends Endocrinol Metab. Oct 2016;27(10):719-730.

28. Hoffman JR, Ratamess NA, Kang J, Falvo MJ, Faigenbaum AD. Effect of protein intake on strength, body composition and endocrine changes in strength/power athletes. J. Int. Soc. Sports Nutr. Jan 1 2006;3:12-18.

29. Howard-Jones PA. Neuroscience and education: myths and messages. Nat. Rev. Neurosci. Dec 2014;15(12):817-824.

30. Hilder TL, Baer LA, Fuller PM, et al. Insulin-independent pathways mediating glucose uptake in hindlimb-suspended skeletal muscle. J Appl Physiol. 2005;99(6):2181-2188.

31. Impey SG, Hearris MA, Hammond KM, et al. Fuel for the Work Required: A Theoretical Framework for Carbohydrate Periodization and the Glycogen Threshold Hypothesis. Sports Med. May 2018;48(5):1031-1048.

32. Kalman DS, Feldman S, Martinez M, Krieger DR, Tallon MJ. Effect of protein source and resistance training on body composition and sex hormones. J. Int. Soc. Sports Nutr. 2007;4(4).

33. Kenny GP, Notley SR, Gagnon D. Direct calorimetry: a brief historical review of its use in the study of human metabolism and thermoregulation. Eur. J. Appl. Physiol. Sep 2017;117(9):1765-1785.

34. Kerksick CM, Arent S, Schoenfeld BJ, et al. International society of sports nutrition position stand: nutrient timing. J. Int. Soc. Sports Nutr. 2017;14:33.

35. Kreider RB, Wilborn CD, Taylor L, et al. ISSN exercise & sport nutrition review: research & recommendations. J. Int. Soc. Sports Nutr. Jan 1 2010;7:7.

36. Krieger JW, Sitren HS, Daniels MJ, Langkamp-Henken B. Effects of variation in protein and carbohydrate intake on body mass and composition during energy restriction: a meta-regression 1. The American journal of clinical nutrition. Feb 1 2006;83(2):260-274.

37. Lam YY, Ravussin E. Analysis of energy metabolism in humans: A review of methodologies. Mol Metab. Nov 2016;5(11):1057-1071.

38. Leroy F, Cofnas N. Should dietary guidelines recommend low red meat intake? Crit Rev Food Sci Nutr. Sep 5 2019:1-10.

39. Millen BE, Lichtenstein AH. USDA Scientific Report of the 2015 Dietary Guidelines Advisory Committee Advisory Report to the Secretary of Health and Human Services and the Secretary of Agriculture. In: Millen BE, Lichtenstein AH, eds2015.

40. Pasiakos SM, Agarwal S, Lieberman HR, Fulgoni VL. Sources and Amounts of Animal, Dairy, and Plant Protein Intake of US Adults in 2007-2010. Nutrients. 2015;7(8):7058-7069.

41. Phillips SM, Fulgoni VL, 3rd, Heaney RP, Nicklas TA, Slavin JL, Weaver CM. Commonly consumed protein foods contribute to nutrient intake, diet quality, and nutrient adequacy. Am. J. Clin. Nutr. Apr 29 2015.

42. Phinney SD. Ketogenic diets and physical performance. Nutr. Metab. (Lond.). Aug 17 2004;1(1):2.

43. Porter J, Nguo K, Collins J, et al. Total energy expenditure measured using doubly labeled water compared with estimated energy requirements in older adults: analysis of primary data. Am. J. Clin. Nutr. 2019;110:1353-1361.

44. Power BT, Kiezebrink K, Allan JL, Campbell MK. Development of a behaviour change workplace-based intervention to improve nurses' eating and physical activity. Pilot and Feasibility Studies. 2021;7(1).

45. Rubin R. Backlash over meat dietary recommendations raises questions about corporate ties to nutrition scientists. JAMA. 2020:E1-E4.

46. Schaefer EJ, Gleason JA, Dansinger ML. Dietary fructose and glucose differentially affect lipid and glucose homeostasis. J. Nutr. Jun 2009;139(6):1257S-1262S.

47. Tarnopolsky MA. Gender differences in metabolism; nutrition and supplements. Journal of science and medicine in sport / Sports Medicine Australia. Sep 1 2000;3(3):287-298.

48. Tarnopolsky M. Protein requirements for endurance athletes. Nutrition (Burbank, Los Angeles County, Calif). 2004;20(7-8):662-668.

49. van Vliet S, Burd NA, van Loon LJ. The Skeletal Muscle Anabolic Response to Plant- versus Animal-Based Protein Consumption. J. Nutr. Jul 29 2015.

50. Venables MC, Jeukendrup AE. Endurance training and obesity: effect on substrate metabolism and insulin sensitivity. Med Sci Sports Exerc. Mar 1 2008;40(3):495-502.

51. Venderley AM, Campbell WW. Vegetarian diets : nutritional considerations for athletes. Sports medicine (Auckland, NZ). 2006;36(4):293-305.

52. Volek JS. Influence of nutrition on responses to resistance training. Med. Sci. Sports Exerc. Apr 1 2004;36(4):689-696

53. Volek JS, Sharman MJ, Forsythe CE. Modification of lipoproteins by very low-carbohydrate diets. J. Nutr. Jun 1 2005;135(6):1339-1342.

54. Volek JS, Sharman MJ. Ch. 29, Diet and Hormonal Responses: Potential Impact on Body Composition. The Endocrine System in Sports and Exercise. May 7 2005:1-18.

55. Volek JS, Westman EC. Very-low-carbohydrate weight-loss diets revisited. Cleve. Clin. J. Med. Nov 1 2002;69(11):849, 853, 856-848 passim.

56. Young VR, Pellet PL. Plant proteins in relation to human and amino acid nutrition. Am. J. Clin. Nutr. 1994;59(Suppl):1203S-1212S.

I need a Remedy...

1. Astrup A, Grunwald GK, Melanson EL, Saris WH, Hill JO. The role of low-fat diets in body weight control: a meta-analysis of ad libitum dietary intervention studies. International journal of obesity and related metabolic disorders : journal of the International Association for the Study of Obesity. 2000;24(12):1545-52.

2. Atkinson FS, Foster-Powell K, Brand-Miller JC. International tables of glycemic index and glycemic load values: 2008. Diabetes Care. 2008;31(12):2281-3. Epub 20081003. doi: 10.2337/dc08-1239.

3. Augustin LSA, Kendall CWC, Jenkins DJA, Willett WC, Astrup A, Barclay AW, et al. Glycemic index, glycemic load and glycemic response: An International Scientific Consensus Summit from the International Carbohydrate Quality Consortium (ICQC). Nutr Metab Cardiovasc Dis. 2015;25(9):795-815. Epub 20150516. doi: 10.1016/j.numecd.2015.05.005.

4. Barclay AW, Petocz P, McMillan-Price J, Flood VM, Prvan T, Mitchell P, et al. Glycemic index, glycemic load, and chronic disease risk--a meta-analysis of observational studies. The American journal of clinical nutrition. 2008;87(3):627-37.

5. Barsby JP, Cowley JM, Leemaqz SY, Grieger JA, McKeating DR, Perkins AV, et al. Nutritional properties of selected superfood extracts and their potential health benefits. PeerJ. 2021;9:e12525. Epub 20211126. doi: 10.7717/peerj.12525.

6. Bhandari P, Sapra A. Low Fat Diet https://www.ncbi.nlm.nih.gov/books/NBK553097/: StatPearls Publishing; 2024 [cited 2024].

7. Brehm BJ, Seeley RJ, Daniels SR, D'Alessio DA. A randomized trial comparing a very low carbohydrate diet and a calorie-restricted low-fat diet on body weight and cardiovascular risk factors in healthy women. The Journal of clinical endocrinology and metabolism. 2003;88(4):1617-23.

8. Calton JB. Prevalence of micronutrient deficiency in popular diet plans. J Int Soc Sports Nutr. 2010;7:24. Epub 20100610. doi: 10.1186/1550-2783-7-24.

9. Carvalho-Peixoto J, Moura MR, Cunha FA, Lollo PC, Monteiro WD, Carvalho LM, et al. Consumption of acai (Euterpe oleracea Mart.) functional beverage reduces muscle stress and improves effort tolerance in elite athletes: a randomized controlled intervention study. Appl Physiol Nutr Metab. 2015;40(7):725-33. doi: 10.1139/apnm-2014-0518.

10. Chen YJ, Wong SHS, Chan COW, Wong CK, Lam CW, Siu PMF. Effects of glycemic index meal and CHO-electrolyte drink on cytokine response and run performance in endurance athletes. Journal of science and medicine in sport / Sports Medicine Australia. 2009;12(6):697-703. doi: 10.1016/j.jsams.2008.05.007.

11. Clark JE. An overview of the contribution of fatness and fitness factors, and the role of exercise, in the formation of health status for individuals who are overweight. J Diabetes Metab Disord. 2012;11(1):19. doi: 10.1186/2251-6581-11-19.

12. Clark JE. Metabolism and nutrition: integration of concepts in a holistic approach to teaching metabolism. HAPS Educator. 2021;25(2):82-102. doi: 10.21692/haps.2021.026.

13. Cobos A, Diaz O. 'Superfoods': Reliability of the Information for Consumers Available on the Web. Foods. 2023;12(3). Epub 20230126. doi: 10.3390/foods12030546.

14. Coyle EF, Jeukendrup AE, Oseto MC, Hodgkinson BJ, Zderic TW. Low-fat diet alters intramuscular substrates and reduces lipolysis and fat oxidation during exercise. Am J Physiol Endocrinol Metab. 2001;280(3):E391-8.

15. Davis JN, Alexander KE, Ventura EE, Kelly LA, Lane CJ, Byrd-Williams CE, et al. Associations of dietary sugar and glycemic index with adiposity and insulin dynamics in overweight Latino youth. Am J Clin Nutr. 2007;86(5):1331-8.

16. Downer S, Berkowitz SA, Harlan TS, Olstad DL, Mozaffarian D. Food is medicine: actions to integrate food and nutrition into healthcare. BMJ. 2020;369:m2482. Epub 20200629. doi: 10.1136/bmj.m2482.

17. Doyle J, Alsan M, Skelley N, Lu Y, Cawley J. Effect of an intensive food-as-medicine program on health and health care use. A random clinical trial. JAMA Intern Med. 2024;184(2):154-63. doi: 10.1001/jamainternmed.2023.6670.

18. Ebbeling CB, Leidig MM, Feldman HA, Lovesky MM, Ludwig DS. Effects of a low-glycemic load vs low-fat diet in obese young adults: a randomized trial. J Am Med Assoc. 2007;297(19):2092-102. doi: 10.1001/jama.297.19.2092.

19. El Assar M, Alvarez-Bustos A, Sosa P, Angulo J, Rodriguez-Manas L. Effect of Physical Activity/Exercise on Oxidative Stress and Inflammation in Muscle and Vascular Aging. Int J Mol Sci. 2022;23(15). Epub 20220805. doi: 10.3390/ijms23158713.

20. Fernández-Ríos A, Laso J, Hoehn D, Amo-Setién FJ, Abajas-Bustillo R, Ortego C, et al. A critical review of superfoods from a holistic nutritional and environmental approach. Journal of Cleaner Production. 2022;379. doi: 10.1016/j.jclepro.2022.134491.

21. Filippou CD, Tsioufis CP, Thomopoulos CG, Mihas CC, Dimitriadis KS, Sotiropoulou LI, et al. Dietary Approaches to Stop Hypertension (DASH) Diet and Blood Pressure Reduction in Adults with and without Hypertension: A

Systematic Review and Meta-Analysis of Randomized Controlled Trials. Adv Nutr. 2020;11(5):1150-60. doi: 10.1093/advances/nmaa041.
22. Franco Lucas B, Alberto Vieira Costa J, Brunner TA. How Information on Superfoods Changes Consumers' Attitudes: An Explorative Survey Study. Foods. 2022;11(13). Epub 20220624. doi: 10.3390/foods11131363.
23. Fratianni A, D'Agostino A, Niro S, Bufano A, Paura B, Panfili G. Loss or Gain of Lipophilic Bioactive Compounds in Vegetables after Domestic Cooking? Effect of Steaming and Boiling. Foods. 2021;10(5). Epub 20210428. doi: 10.3390/foods10050960.
24. Freeland-Graves JH, Nitzke S, Academy of N, Dietetics. Position of the academy of nutrition and dietetics: total diet approach to healthy eating. J Acad Nutr Diet. 2013;113(2):307-17. doi: 10.1016/j.jand.2012.12.013.
25. Fusco D, Colloca G, Lo Monaco MR, Cesari M. Effects of antioxidant supplementation on the aging process. Clinical Investigation in Aging. 2007;2(3):377-87.
26. Kampa M, Nifli A-P, Notas G, Castanas E. Polyphenols and cancer cell growth. Reviews of physiology, biochemistry and pharmacology. 2007;159:79-113. doi: 10.1007/112_2006_0702.
27. Kerksick CM, Arent S, Schoenfeld BJ, Stout JR, Campbell B, Wilborn CD, et al. International society of sports nutrition position stand: nutrient timing. J Int Soc Sports Nutr. 2017;14:33. doi: 10.1186/s12970-017-0189-4.
28. Kumar SV, Saritha G, Fareedullah M. Role of antioxidants and oxidative stress in cardiovascular diseases. Ann Biol Res. 2010;1(3):158-73.
29. La Berge AF. How the ideology of low-fat conquered America. J Hist Med Allied Sci. 2008;63(2):139-77. Epub 20080223. doi: 10.1093/jhmas/jrn001.
30. Lee CD, Hardin CC, Longo DL, Ingelfinger JR. Nutrition in Medicine - A New Review Article Series. N Eng J Med. 2024;390(14):1324-5. doi: 10.1056/NEJMe2313282.
31. Livesey G, Taylor R, Livesey HF, Buyken AE, Jenkins DJA, Augustin LSA, et al. Dietary Glycemic Index and Load and the Risk of Type 2 Diabetes: Assessment of Causal Relations. Nutrients. 2019;11(6). Epub 20190625. doi: 10.3390/nu11061436.
32. Lobo V, Patil A, Phatak A, Chandra N. Free radicals, antioxidants and functional foods: Impact on human health. Pharmacogn Rev. 2010;4(8):118-26. doi: 10.4103/0973-7847.70902.
33. Mason SA, Trewin AJ, Parker L, Wadley GD. Antioxidant supplements and endurance exercise: Current evidence and mechanistic insights. Redox Biol. 2020:101471. doi: 10.1016/j.redox.2020.101471.
34. McMaster MW, Sharma D, Kafle P, Frishman WH, Aronow WS. Use of the DASH diet and coronary artery disease. Cardiol Rev. 2024;32(2):153-6. doi: 10.1097/CRD.0000000000000482.
35. Mirza NM, Palmer MG, Sinclair KB, McCarter R, He J, Ebbeling CB, et al. Effects of a low glycemic load or a low-fat dietary intervention on body weight in obese Hispanic American children and adolescents: a randomized controlled trial. The American journal of clinical nutrition. 2013;97(2):276-85. doi: 10.3945/ajcn.112.042630.
36. Munoz ME, Galan AI, Palacios E, Diez MA, Muguerza B, Cobaleda C, et al. Effect of an antioxidant functional food beverage on exercise-induced oxidative stress: a long-term and large-scale clinical intervention study. Toxicology. 2010;278(1):101-11. doi: 10.1016/j.tox.2009.10.015.
37. Nogiec CD, Kasif S. To supplement or not to supplement: a metabolic network framework for human nutritional supplements. PLoS One. 2013;8(8):e68751. doi: 10.1371/journal.pone.0068751.
38. Onwuzo C, Olukorode JO, Omokore OA, Odunaike OS, Omiko R, Osaghae OW, et al. DASH Diet: A Review of Its Scientifically Proven Hypertension Reduction and Health Benefits. Cureus. 2023;15(9):e44692. Epub 20230904. doi: 10.7759/cureus.44692.
39. Ristow M, Zarse K, Oberbach A, Klöting N, Birringer M, Kiehntopf M, et al. Antioxidants prevent health-promoting effects of physical exercise in humans. Proc Natl Acad Sci U S A. 2009;106(21):8665-70. doi: 10.1073/pnas.0903485106.
40. Rodriguez-Bies E, Santa-Cruz Calvo S, Navas P, Lopez-Lluch G. Resveratrol: An ergogenic compound. Revista Andaluza de Medicina del Deporte. 2009;2(1):12-8.
41. Rouhani MH, Kelishadi R, Hashemipour M, Esmaillzadeh A, Azadbakht L. The effect of low glycemic index diet on body weight status and blood pressure in overweight adolescent girls: a randomized clinical trial. Nutr Res Pract. 2013;7(5):385-92. doi: 10.4162/nrp.2013.7.5.385.
42. Saper RB, Eisenberg DM, Phillips RS. Common dietary supplements for weight loss. Am Fam Physician. 2004;70:1731-8.
43. Sedlacek SM, Playdon MC, Wolfe P, Mcginley JN, Wisthoff MR, Daeninck EA, et al. Effect of a low fat versus a low carbohydrate weight loss dietary intervention on biomarkers of long term survival in breast cancer patients ('CHOICE'): study protocol. BMC Cancer. 2011;11:287.
44. Stein CM. Are herbal products dietary supplements or drugs? An important question for public safety. Clin Pharmacol Ther. 2002;71(6):411-3.
45. Theodoridis X, Chourdakis M, Chrysoula L, Chroni V, Tirodimos I, Dipla K, et al. Adherence to the DASH Diet and Risk of Hypertension: A Systematic Review and Meta-Analysis. Nutrients. 2023;15(14). Epub 20230724. doi: 10.3390/nu15143261.
46. Vega-Lopez S, Venn BJ, Slavin JL. Relevance of the Glycemic Index and Glycemic Load for Body Weight, Diabetes, and Cardiovascular Disease. Nutrients. 2018;10(10). doi: 10.3390/nu10101361.
47. Volek JS, Kackley ML, Buga A. Nutritional Considerations During Major Weight Loss Therapy: Focus on Optimal Protein and a Low-Carbohydrate Dietary Pattern. Curr Nutr Rep. 2024. Epub 20240530. doi: 10.1007/s13668-024-00548-6.
48. Yuzbashian E, Asghari G, Mirmiran P, Amouzegar-Bahambari P, Azizi F. Adherence to low-sodium Dietary Approaches to Stop Hypertension-style diet may decrease the risk of incident chronic kidney disease among high-risk patients: a secondary prevention in prospective cohort study. Nephrol Dial Transplant. 2018;33(7):1159-68. doi: 10.1093/ndt/gfx352.

Carbs … we don't need no stinking Carbs…

1. Andrikopoulos S. The Paleo diet and diabetes. Med J Aust. 2016;205(4):151-2. doi: 10.5694/mja16.00347.
2. Bortolotti M, Kreis R, Debard C, Cariou B, Faeh D, Chetiveaux M, et al. High protein intake reduces intrahepatocellular lipid deposition in humans. The American journal of clinical nutrition. 2009;90(4):1002-10. doi: 10.3945/ajcn.2008.27296.
3. Bostock ECS, Kirkby KC, Taylor BV, Hawrelak JA. Consumer Reports of "Keto Flu" Associated With the Ketogenic Diet. Front Nutr. 2020;7:20. doi: 10.3389/fnut.2020.00020.
4. Brand-Miller JC, Griffin HJ, Colagiuri S. The carnivore connection hypothesis: revisited. J Obes. 2012;2012:258624. Epub 20111222. doi: 10.1155/2012/258624.
5. Brown MR, Klish WJ, Hollander J, Campbell MA, Forbes GB. A high protein, low calorie liquid diet in the treatment of very obese adolescents: long-term effect on lean body mass. The American journal of clinical nutrition. 1983;38(1):20-31.
6. Burke LM, Ross ML, Garvican-Lewis LA, Welvaert M, Heikura IA, Forbes SG, et al. Low carbohydrate, high fat diet impairs exercise economy and negates the performance benefit from intensified training in elite race walkers. J Physiol. 2017;595(9):2785-807. doi: 10.1113/JP273230.
7. Calton JB. Prevalence of micronutrient deficiency in popular diet plans. J Int Soc Sports Nutr. 2010;7:24. Epub 20100610. doi: 10.1186/1550-2783-7-24.
8. Cambeses-Franco C, González-García S, Feijoo G, Moreira MT. Is the Paleo diet safe for health and the environment? Sci Total Environ. 2021;781. doi: 10.1016/j.scitotenv.2021.146717.
9. Cassady BA, Charboneau NL, Brys EE, Crouse KA, Beitz DC, Wilson T. Effects of low carbohydrate diets high in red meats or poultry, fish and shellfish on plasma lipids and weight loss. Nutr Metab (Lond). 2007;4:23. Epub 20071031. doi: 10.1186/1743-7075-4-23.
10. De Chiara F, Ureta Checcllo C, Ramon Azcon J. High Protein Diet and Metabolic Plasticity in Non-Alcoholic Fatty Liver Disease: Myths and Truths. Nutrients. 2019;11(12). Epub 20191206. doi: 10.3390/nu11122985.
11. Demol S, Yackobovitch-Gavan M, Shalitin S, Nagelberg N, Gillon-Keren M, Phillip M. Low-carbohydrate (low & high-fat) versus high-carbohydrate low-fat diets in the treatment of obesity in adolescents. Acta Paediatr. 2009;98(2):346-51. doi: doi: 10.1111/j.1651-2227.2008.01051.
12. Dyson PA. A review of low and reduced carbohydrate diets and weight loss in type 2 diabetes. J Hum Nutr Diet. 2008;21(6):530-8. doi: 10.1111/j.1365-277X.2008.00896.x.
13. Fenton TR, Fenton CJ. Paleo diet still lacks evidence. Am J Clin Nutr. 2016;104(3):844. doi: 10.3945/ajcn.116.139006.
14. Friedman JM, Halaas JL. Leptin and the regulation of body weight in mammals. Nature. 1998;395(6704):763-70.
15. Gately PJ, King NA, Greatwood HC, Humphrey LC, Radley D, Cooke CB, et al. Does a high-protein diet improve weight loss in overweight and obese children? Obesity (Silver Spring). 2007;15(6):1527-34. doi: 10.1038/oby.2007.181.
16. Harvey KL, Holcomb LE, Kolwicz SC, Jr. Ketogenic Diets and Exercise Performance. Nutrients. 2019;11(10). doi: 10.3390/nu11102296.
17. Hoffman JR, Ratamess NA, Kang J, Falvo MJ, Faigenbaum AD. Effect of protein intake on strength, body composition and endocrine changes in strength/power athletes. J Int Soc Sports Nutr. 2006;3:12-8. doi: 10.1186/1550-2783-3-2-12.
18. Kirkpatrick CF, Bolick JP, Kris-Etherton PM, Sikand G, Aspry KE, Soffer DE, et al. Review of current evidence and clinical recommendations on the effects of low-carbohydrate and very-low-carbohydrate (including ketogenic) diets for the management of body weight and other cardiometabolic risk factors: A scientific statement from the National Lipid Association Nutrition and Lifestyle Task Force. J Clin Lipidol. 2019;13(5):689-711 e1. Epub 20190913. doi: 10.1016/j.jacl.2019.08.003.
19. Ko GJ, Rhee CM, Kalantar-Zadeh K, Joshi S. The Effects of High-Protein Diets on Kidney Health and Longevity. J Am Soc Nephrol. 2020;31(8):1667-79. Epub 20200715. doi: 10.1681/ASN.2020010028.
20. Koopman R, Saris WHM, Wagenmakers AJM, van Loon LJC. Nutritional interventions to promote post-exercise muscle protein synthesis. Sports Med. 2007;37(10):895-906.
21. Krebs NF, Gao D, Gralla J, Collins JS, Johnson SL. Efficacy and safety of a high protein, low carbohydrate diet for weight loss in severely obese adolescents. The Journal of pediatrics. 2010;157(2):252-8. doi: 10.1016/j.jpeds.2010.02.010.
22. Lennerz BS, Mey JT, Henn OH, Ludwig DS. Behavioral Characteristics and Self-Reported Health Status among 2029 Adults Consuming a "Carnivore Diet". Current Developments in Nutrition. 2021;5:nzab133. doi: 10.1093/cdn/nzab133.
23. Leroy F, Cofnas N. Should dietary guidelines recommend low red meat intake? Crit Rev Food Sci Nutr. 2019:1-10. doi: 10.1080/10408398.2019.1657063.
24. Manninen AH. Are high-protein diets safe for kidney function? J Am Diet Assoc. 2007;107(10):1722; author reply doi: 10.1016/j.jada.2007.08.020.
25. Manheimer EW, van Zuuren EJ, Fedorowicz Z, Pijl H. Paleolithic nutrition for metabolic syndrome: systematic review and meta-analysis. Am J Clin Nutr. 2015;102(4):922-32. Epub 20150812. doi: 10.3945/ajcn.115.113613.
26. Nylen K, Likhodii S, Burnham WM. The ketogenic diet: proposed mechanisms of action. NURT. 2009;6(2):402-5. doi: 10.1016/j.nurt.2009.01.021.
27. O'Hearn A. Can a carnivore diet provide all essential nutrients? Curr Opin Endocrinol Diabetes Obes. 2020;27(5):312-6. doi: 10.1097/MED.0000000000000576..
28. O'Hearn A. A survey of improvements experienced on a carnivore diet compared to only carbohydrate restriction 2019.

29.	Paoli A, Bianco A, Grimaldi KA. The Ketogenic Diet and Sport. Exerc Sport Sci Rev. 2015;43(3):153-62. doi: 10.1249/JES.0000000000000050.
30.	Paoli A, Grimaldi K, D'Agostino D, Cenci L, Moro T, Bianco A, et al. Ketogenic diet does not affect strength performance in elite artistic gymnasts. J Int Soc Sports Nutr. 2012;9(1):34. doi: 10.1186/1550-2783-9-34.
31.	Paoli A, Rubini A, Volek JS, Grimaldi KA. Beyond weight loss: a review of the therapeutic uses of very-low-carbohydrate (ketogenic) diets. Eur J Clin Nutr. 2013;67(8):789-96. doi: 10.1038/ejcn.2013.116.
32.	Phillips SM. Dietary protein for athletes: from requirements to metabolic advantage. Applied physiology, nutrition, and metabolism = Physiologie appliquée, nutrition et métabolisme. 2006;31(6):647-54. doi: 10.1139/h06-035.
33.	Pilis K, Pilis A, Stec K, Pilis W, Langfort J, Letkiewicz S, et al. Three-Year Chronic Consumption of Low-Carbohydrate Diet Impairs Exercise Performance and Has a Small Unfavorable Effect on Lipid Profile in Middle-Aged Men. Nutrients. 2018;10(12). doi: 10.3390/nu10121914.
34.	Pinckaers PJ, Churchward-Venne TA, Bailey D, van Loon LJ. Ketone Bodies and Exercise Performance: The Next Magic Bullet or Merely Hype? Sports Med. 2017;47(3):383-91. doi: 10.1007/s40279-016-0577-y.
35.	Pitt C. Cutting through the Paleo hype: The evidence for the Paleolithic diet. Aust Fam Physician. 2016;45(1):35-8.
36.	Protogerou C, Leroy F, Hagger MS. Beliefs and Experiences of Individuals Following a Zero-Carb Diet. Behav Sci (Basel). 2021;11(12). Epub 20211123. doi: 10.3390/bs11120161.
37.	Tarantino G, Citro V, Finelli C. Hype or Reality: Should Patients with Metabolic Syndrome-related NAFLD be on the Hunter-Gatherer (Paleo) Diet to Decrease Morbidity? J Gastrointestin Liver Dis. 2015;24(3):359-68. doi: 10.15403/jgld.2014.1121.243.gta.
38.	Volek JS, Westman EC. Very-low-carbohydrate weight-loss diets revisited. Cleve Clin J Med. 2002;69(11):849, 53, 56-8 passim. doi: 10.3949/ccjm.69.11.849.
39.	Volek JS, Sharman MJ, Forsythe CE. Modification of lipoproteins by very low-carbohydrate diets. J Nutr. 2005;135(6):1339-42.
40.	Volek JS, Kackley ML, Buga A. Nutritional Considerations During Major Weight Loss Therapy: Focus on Optimal Protein and a Low-Carbohydrate Dietary Pattern. Curr Nutr Rep. 2024. Epub 20240530. doi: 10.1007/s13668-024-00548-6.
41.	Westman EC, Feinman RD, Mavropoulos JC, Vernon MC, Volek JS, Wortman JA, et al. Low-carbohydrate nutrition and metabolism. The American journal of clinical nutrition. 2007;86(2):276-84. doi: 10.1093/ajcn/86.2.276.

Old McDonald had a farm...

1.	United States Food and Drug Administration. Environment and Contaminants: Chemicals in Food. America's Children and the Environment. Third ed. 2019.
2.	United States Department of Agriculture. USDA Agricultural Marketing Service https://www.ams.usda.gov/grades-standards/organic-standards: U.S. Department of Agriculture; 2024 [cited 2024].
3.	Annuziata A, Mariani A. Consumer perception of sustainability attributes in organic and local food. Recent Pat Food Nutr Agric. 2018;9(2):87-96. doi: 10.2174/2212798410666171215112058.
4.	Bhagavathula AS, Vidyasagar K, Khubchandani J. Organic Food Consumption and Risk of Obesity: A Systematic Review and Meta-Analysis. Healthcare (Basel). 2022;10(2). Epub 20220126. doi: 10.3390/healthcare10020231.
5.	Crinnion WJ. Organic foods contain higher levels of certain nutrients, lower levels of pesticides, and may provide health benefits for the consumer. Altern Med Rev. 2010;15(1):4-12.
6.	de Araujo-Ramos AT, Passoni MT, Romano MA, Romano RM, Martino-Andrade AJ. Controversies on Endocrine and Reproductive Effects of Glyphosate and Glyphosate-Based Herbicides: A Mini-Review. Front Endocrinol (Lausanne). 2021;12:627210. Epub 20210315. doi: 10.3389/fendo.2021.627210.
7.	Fritsche K, Zikova-Kloas A, Marx-Stoelting P, Braeuning A. Metabolism-Disrupting Chemicals Affecting the Liver: Screening, Testing, and Molecular Pathway Identification. Int J Mol Sci. 2023;24(3). Epub 20230131. doi: 10.3390/ijms24032686.
8.	Glibowski P. Organic food and health. Rocz Panstw Zakl Hig. 2020;71(2):131-6. doi: 10.32394/rpzh.2020.0110.
9.	Karami-Mohajeri S, Abdollahi M. Toxic influence of organophosphate, carbamate, and organochlorine pesticides on cellular metabolism of lipids, proteins, and carbohydrates: a systematic review. Hum Exp Toxicol. 2011;30(9):1119-40. Epub 20101111. doi: 10.1177/0960327110388959.
10.	La Merrill MA, Vandenberg LN, Smith MT, Goodson W, Browne P, Patisaul HB, et al. Consensus on the key characteristics of endocrine-disrupting chemicals as a basis for hazard identification. Nat Rev Endocrinol. 2020;16(1):45-57. Epub 20191112. doi: 10.1038/s41574-019-0273-8.
11.	Marraudino M, Bonaldo B, Farinetti A, Panzica G, Ponti G, Gotti S. Metabolism Disrupting Chemicals and Alteration of Neuroendocrine Circuits Controlling Food Intake and Energy Metabolism. Front Endocrinol (Lausanne). 2018;9:766. Epub 20190109. doi: 10.3389/fendo.2018.00766.
12.	McEvoy M. Organic 101: What the USDA Organic Label means https://www.usda.gov/media/blog/2012/03/22/organic-101-what-usda-organic-label-means: U.S. Department of Agriculture; 2012 [cited 2024]. https://www.usda.gov/media/blog/2012/03/22/organic-101-what-usda-organic-label-means].
13.	Oteng AB, Kersten S. Mechanisms of Action of trans Fatty Acids. Adv Nutr. 2020;11(3):697-708. doi: 10.1093/advances/nmz125.
14.	Peillex C, Pelletier M. The impact and toxicity of glyphosate and glyphosate-based herbicides on health and immunity. J Immunotoxicol. 2020;17(1):163-74. doi: 10.1080/1547691X.2020.1804492.

15. Schafer KS, Kegley SE. Persistent toxic chemicals in the US food supply. J Epidemiol Community Health. 2002;56:813-7.
16. Strassner C, Cavoski I, Di Cagno R, Kahl J, Kesse-Guyot E, Lairon D, et al. How the Organic Food System Supports Sustainable Diets and Translates These into Practice. Front Nutr. 2015;2:19. Epub 20150629. doi: 10.3389/fnut.2015.00019.
17. Vardakas P, Veskoukis AS, Rossiou D, Gournikis C, Kapetanopoulou T, Karzi V, et al. A Mixture of Endocrine Disruptors and the Pesticide Roundup((R)) Induce Oxidative Stress in Rabbit Liver When Administered under the Long-Term Low-Dose Regimen: Reinforcing the Notion of Real-Life Risk Simulation. Toxics. 2022;10(4). Epub 20220414. doi: 10.3390/toxics10040190.
18. Vigar V, Myers S, Oliver C, Arellano J, Robinson S, Leifert C. A Systematic Review of Organic Versus Conventional Food Consumption: Is There a Measurable Benefit on Human Health? Nutrients. 2019;12(1). Epub 20191218. doi: 10.3390/nu12010007

Everywhere you go, there we are…

1. Beaulieu DA, Best LA. Eat, pray, love: disordered eating in religious and non-religious men and women. J Eat Disord. 2022;10(1):198. Epub 20221220. doi: 10.1186/s40337-022-00721-8.
2. Bruss MB, Applegate B, Quitugua J, Palacios RT, Morris JR. Ethnicity and diet of children: development of culturally sensitive measures. Health Educ Behav. 2007;34(5):735-47. Epub 20070207. doi: 10.1177/1090198106294648.
3. Caprara G. Mediterranean-Type Dietary Pattern and Physical Activity: The Winning Combination to Counteract the Rising Burden of Non-Communicable Diseases (NCDs). Nutrients. 2021;13(2). Epub 20210128. doi: 10.3390/nu13020429.
4. Chouraqui JP, Turck D, Briend A, Darmaun D, Bocquet A, Feillet F, et al. Religious dietary rules and their potential nutritional and health consequences. Int J Epidemiol. 2021;50(1):12-26. doi: 10.1093/ije/dyaa182.
5. Clark JE. An overview of the contribution of fatness and fitness factors, and the role of exercise, in the formation of health status for individuals who are overweight. J Diabetes Metab Disord. 2012;11(1):19. doi: 10.1186/2251-6581-11-19.
6. Clark JE. Diets and Diet Therapy: Diet Supplements for Exercise. In: Ferranti P, Berry EM, Anderson JR, editors. Encyclopedia of Food Security and Sustainability. 2: Elsevier; 2019. p. 161-70.
7. Clark JE. Metabolism and nutrition: integration of concepts in a holistic approach to teaching metabolism. HAPS Educator. 2021;25(2):82-102. doi: 10.21692/haps.2021.026.
8. Diolintzi A, Panagiotakos DB, Sidossis LS. From Mediterranean diet to Mediterranean lifestyle: a narrative review. Public Health Nutr. 2019;22(14):2703-13. Epub 20190603. doi: 10.1017/S1368980019000612. PubMed PMID: 31156076; PubMed Central PMCID: PMCPMC10260601.
9. Guasch-Ferre M, Willett WC. The Mediterranean diet and health: a comprehensive overview. J Intern Med. 2021;290(3):549-66. Epub 20210823. doi: 10.1111/joim.13333. PubMed PMID: 34423871.
10. James DC. Factors influencing food choices, dietary intake, and nutrition-related attitudes among African Americans: application of a culturally sensitive model. Ethn Health. 2004;9(4):349-67. doi:10.1080/1355785042000285375.
11. Keys A. Mediterranean diet and public health: Personal reflections. The American Journal of Clinical Nutrition. 1995;61(6):1321S.
12. Kuehn BM. Heritage diets and culturally appropriate dietary advice may help combat chronic diseases. JAMA. 2019;322(23):2271-3. doi: 10.1001/jama.2019.18431.
13. Lacatusu CM, Grigorescu ED, Floria M, Onofriescu A, Mihai BM. The Mediterranean Diet: From an Environment-Driven Food Culture to an Emerging Medical Prescription. Int J Environ Res Public Health. 2019;16(6). Epub 20190315. doi: 10.3390/ijerph16060942.
14. Lelwica M. The religion of thinness. Scripta Instituti Donneriani Aboensis. 2011;23:257-85. doi: DOI:10.30674/scripta.67400.
15. Martini D. Health Benefits of Mediterranean Diet. Nutrients. 2019;11(8). Epub 20190805. doi:10.3390/nu11081802.
16. Mocciaro G, Ziauddeen N, Godos J, Marranzano M, Chan M-Y, Ray S. Does a Mediterranean-type dietary pattern exert a cardio-protective effect outside the Mediterranean region? A review of current evidence. International Journal of Food Sciences and Nutrition. 2017;69(5):524-35. doi:10.1080/09637486.2017.1391752.
17. Shai I, Schwarzfuchs D, Henkin Y, Shahar DR, Witkow S, Greenberg I, et al. Weight Loss with a Low-Carbohydrate, Mediterranean, or Low-Fat Diet. The New England journal of medicine. 2008;359(3):229-41. doi: 10.1056/NEJMoa0708681.
18. Shatenstein B, Ghadirian P. Influences on diet, health behaviours and their outcome in select ethnocultural and religious groups. Nutrition. 1998;14(2):223-30. doi: 10.1016/50899-9007(97)00425-5.
19. Sibal V. Food: Identity of culture and religion. 2018.
20. Tahreem A, Rakha A, Rabail R, Nazir A, Socol CT, Maerescu CM, et al. Fad Diets: Facts and Fiction. Front Nutr. 2022;9:960922. Epub 20220705. doi: 10.3389/fnut.2022.960922.
21. Wright KE, Lucero JE, Ferguson JK, Granner ML, Devereux PG, Pearson JL, et al. The impact that cultural food security has on identity and well-being in the second-generation U.S. American minority college students. Food Secur. 2021;13(3):701-15. Epub 20210125. doi: 10.1007/s12571-020-01140-w.
22. Zeller BE. Totem and taboo in the grocery store. Quasi-religious foodways in North America. Religion and Food. 2015;26:11-31.
23. Zeller BE, Dallam MW, Neilson RL, Rubel NL. Religion, Food, and Eating in North America. New York, NY: Columbia University Press; 2014. 376 p. ISBN: 978-0-231-53731-5

For every season, a time to eat...

1. Antoni R, Johnston KL, Collins AL, Robertson MD. Intermittent v. continuous energy restriction: differential effects on postprandial glucose and lipid metabolism following matched weight loss in overweight/obese participants. Br. J. Nutr. Mar 2018;119(5):507-516.
2. Chaix A, Zarrinpar A. The effects of time-restricted feeding on lipid metabolism and adiposity. Adipocyte. Oct-Dec 2015;4(4):319-324.
3. Chaix A, Zarrinpar A, Miu P, Panda S. Time-restricted feeding is a preventative and therapeutic intervention against diverse nutritional challenges. Cell Metab. Dec 2 2014;20(6):991-1005.
4. Clark JE. An overview of the contribution of fatness and fitness factors, and the role of exercise, in the formation of health status for individuals who are overweight. J. Diabetes Metab. Disord. Jan 1 2012;11(1):19.
5. Clark JE. Metabolism and nutrition: integration of concepts in a holistic approach to teaching metabolism. HAPS Educator. 2021;25(2):82-102.
6. Di Francesco A, Di Germanio C, Brenier M, de Cabo R. A time to fast. Science. 2018;362:770-775.
7. Garaulet M, Gomez-Abellan P. Timing of food intake and obesity: a novel association. Physiol Behav. Jul 2014;134:44-50.
8. Geer EB, Shen W. Gender differences in insulin resistance, body composition, and energy balance. Gend. Med. Jan 1 2009;6 Suppl 1:60-75.
9. Headland M, Clifton PM, Carter S, Keogh JB. Weight-Loss Outcomes: A Systematic Review and Meta-Analysis of Intermittent Energy Restriction Trials Lasting a Minimum of 6 Months. Nutrients. Jun 8 2016;8(6).
10. Henry CJK. Basal metabolic rate studies in humans: measurement and development of new equations. Public Health Nutr. 2007;8(7a):1133-1152
11. Jéquier E. Leptin signaling, adiposity, and energy balance. Ann. N. Y. Acad. Sci. Jun 1 2002;967:379-388.
12. Keogh JB, Pedersen E, Petersen KS, Clifton PM. Effects of intermittent compared to continuous energy restriction on short-term weight loss and long-term weight loss maintenance. Clin Obes. Jun 2014;4(3):150-156.
13. Kerksick CM, Arent S, Schoenfeld BJ, et al. International society of sports nutrition position stand: nutrient timing. J. Int. Soc. Sports Nutr. 2017;14:33.
14. Lewis DA, Kamon E, Hodgson JL. Physiological differences between genders. Implications for sports conditioning. Sports Med. 1986;3(5):357-369.
15. Loh X, Sun L, Allen JC, et al. Gender differences in fasting and postprandial metabolic traits predictive of subclinical atherosclerosis in an asymptomatic Chinese population. Sci. Rep. Oct 7 2022;12(1):16890.
16. Mancini F, Loucks TL, Cameron JL, Berga SL. Sex steroid milieu does not alter the impact of fasting on eptin levels in women. Fertil. Steril. Dec 2005;84(6):1768-1771.
17. Mattsson C, Rask E, Carlström K, et al. Gender-specific links between hepatic 11beta reduction of cortisone and adipokines. Obesity (Silver Spring). Apr 1 2007;15(4):887-894.
18. Mattson MP, Longo VD, Harvie M. Impact of intermittent fasting on health and disease processes. Ageing Res Rev. Oct 2017;39:46-58.
19. Mittendorfer B, Horowitz JF, Klein S. Gender differences in lipid and glucose kinetics during short-term fasting. Am. J. Physiol. Endocrinol. Metab. 2001;281:E1333-E1339.
20. Ramirez-Zea M. Validation of three predictive equations for basal metabolic rate in adults. Public Health Nutr. Oct 2005;8(7A):1213-1228
21. Rynders CA, Thomas EA, Zaman A, Pan Z, Catenacci VA, Melanson EL. Effectiveness of Intermittent Fasting and Time-Restricted Feeding Compared to Continuous Energy Restriction for Weight Loss. Nutrients. Oct 14 2019;11(10).
22. Seimon RV, Roekenes JA, Zibellini J, et al. Do intermittent diets provide physiological benefits over continuous diets for weight loss? A systematic review of clinical trials. Mol Cell Endocrinol. Dec 15 2015;418 Pt 2:153-172.
23. Soeters MR, Sauerwein HP, Groener JE, et al. Gender-related differences in the metabolic response to fasting. J. Clin. Endocrinol. Metab. Sep 2007;92(9):3646-3652.
24. Tarnopolsky MA. Gender differences in metabolism; nutrition and supplements. Journal of science and medicine in sport / Sports Medicine Australia. Sep 1 2000;3(3):287-298.
25. Tinsley GM, La Bounty PM. Effects of intermittent fasting on body composition and clinical health markers in humans. Nutr. Rev. Oct 2015;73(10):661-674.
26. Varady KA. Intermittent versus daily calorie restriction: which diet regimen is more effective for weight loss? Obes. Rev. Jul 2011;12(7):e593-601.
27. Wei M, Brandhorst S, Shelehchi M, et al. Fasting-mimicking diet and markers/risk factors for aging, diabetes, cancer, and cardiovascular disease. Sci. Transl. Med. Feb 15 2017;9(377).
28. Zandian M, Ioakimidis I, Bergh C, Leon M, Sodersten P. A sex difference in the response to fasting. Physiol. Behav. 2011;103(5):530-534.

Go green or go home...

1. Abraham K, Trefflich I, Gauch F, Weikert C. Nutritional Intake and Biomarker Status in Strict Raw Food Eaters. Nutrients. 2022;14(9). Epub 20220421. doi: 10.3390/nu14091725.
2. American College of Sports Medicine, American Dietetic Association, Dieticians of Canda. Nutrition and Athletic Performance. Med Sci Sports Exerc. 2009. doi: 10.1249/MSS.0b013e318190eb86.
3. Bakaloudi DR, Halloran A, Rippin HL, Oikonomidou AC, Dardavesis TI, Williams J, et al. Intake and adequacy of the vegan diet. A systematic review of the evidence. Clin Nutr. 2021;40(5):3503-21. Epub 20201207. doi: 10.1016/j.clnu.2020.11.035

4. Chan Q, Stamler J, Brown IJ, Daviglus ML, Van Horn L, Dyer AR, et al. Relation of raw and cooked vegetable consumption to blood pressure: the INTERMAP Study. J Hum Hypertens. 2014;28(6):353-9. Epub 20131121. doi: 10.1038/jhh.2013.115.

5. Ciuris C, Lynch HM, Wharton C, Johnston CS. A Comparison of Dietary Protein Digestibility, Based on DIAAS Scoring, in Vegetarian and Non-Vegetarian Athletes. Nutrients. 2019;11(12). doi: 10.3390/nu11123016.

6. Falchetti A, Cavati G, Valenti R, Mingiano C, Cosso R, Gennari L, et al. The effects of vegetarian diets on bone health: A literature review. Front Endocrinol (Lausanne). 2022;13:899375. Epub 20220805. doi: 10.3389/fendo.2022.899375.

7. Haider S, Sima A, Kuhn T, Wakolbinger M. The Association between Vegan Dietary Patterns and Physical Activity-A Cross-Sectional Online Survey. Nutrients. 2023;15(8). Epub 20230412. doi: 10.3390/nu15081847.

8. Jedut P, Glibowski P, Skrzypek M. Comparison of the Health Status of Vegetarians and Omnivores Based on Biochemical Blood Tests, Body Composition Analysis and Quality of Nutrition. Nutrients. 2023;15(13). Epub 20230705. doi: 10.3390/nu15133038.

9. Leroy F, Cofnas N. Should dietary guidelines recommend low red meat intake? Crit Rev Food Sci Nutr. 2019:1-10. doi: 10.1080/10408398.2019.1657063.

10. Mariotti F, Gardner CD. Dietary Protein and Amino Acids in Vegetarian Diets-A Review. Nutrients. 2019;11(11). Epub 20191104. doi: 10.3390/nu11112661.

11. Neufingerl N, Eilander A. Nutrient Intake and Status in Adults Consuming Plant-Based Diets Compared to Meat-Eaters: A Systematic Review. Nutrients. 2021;14(1). Epub 20211223. doi: 10.3390/nu14010029.

12. Neufingerl N, Eilander A. Nutrient Intake and Status in Children and Adolescents Consuming Plant-Based Diets Compared to Meat-Eaters: A Systematic Review. Nutrients. 2023;15(20). Epub 20231011. doi: 10.3390/nu15204341.

13. Pahlavani N, Azizi-Soleiman F. The effects of a raw vegetarian diet from a clinical perspective; review of the available evidence. Clinical Nutrition Open Science. 2023;49:107-12. doi: 10.1016/j.nutos.2023.04.001.

14. Petroski W, Minich DM. Is There Such a Thing as "Anti-Nutrients"? A Narrative Review of Perceived Problematic Plant Compounds. Nutrients. 2020;12(10). Epub 20200924. doi: 10.3390/nu12102929.

15. Rogerson D. Vegan diets: practical advice for athletes and exercisers. J Int Soc Sports Nutr. 2017;14:36. Epub 20170913. doi: 10.1186/s12970-017-0192-9.

16. Rumm-Kreuter D, Demmel I. Comparison of vitamin losses in vegetables due to various cooking methods. Journal of Nutritional Science and Vitaminology. 1990;36(4-Supplement):S7-S15.

17. Sakkas H, Bozidis P, Touzios C, Kolios D, Athanasiou G, Athanasopoulou E, et al. Nutritional Status and the Influence of the Vegan Diet on the Gut Microbiota and Human Health. Medicina (Kaunas). 2020;56(2). Epub 20200222. doi: 10.3390/medicina56020088.

18. Tahreem A, Rakha A, Rabail R, Nazir A, Socol CT, Maerescu CM, et al. Fad Diets: Facts and Fiction. Front Nutr. 2022;9:960922. Epub 20220705. doi: 10.3389/fnut.2022.960922.

19. Tso R, Forde CG. Unintended Consequences: Nutritional Impact and Potential Pitfalls of Switching from Animal- to Plant-Based Foods. Nutrients. 2021;13(8). Epub 20210723. doi: 10.3390/nu13082527.

20. van Vliet S, Burd NA, van Loon LJ. The Skeletal Muscle Anabolic Response to Plant- versus Animal-Based Protein Consumption. J Nutr. 2015. doi: 10.3945/jn.114.204305.

21. Venderley AM, Campbell WW. Vegetarian diets : nutritional considerations for athletes. Sports medicine (Auckland, NZ). 2006;36(4):293-305.

22. Wang T, Masedunskas A, Willett WC, Fontana L. Vegetarian and vegan diets: benefits and drawbacks. Eur Heart J. 2023;44(36):3423-39. doi: 10.1093/eurheartj/ehad436.

23. West S, Monteyne AJ, van der Heijden I, Stephens FB, Wall BT. Nutritional Considerations for the Vegan Athlete. Adv Nutr. 2023;14(4):774-95. Epub 20230429. doi: 10.1016/j.advnut.2023.04.012.

24. Williams E, Vardavoulia A, Lally P, Gardner B. Experiences of initiating and maintaining a vegan diet among young adults: A qualitative study. Appetite. 2023;180:106357. Epub 20221029. doi:10.1016/j.appet.2022.106357.

25. Abraham K, Trefflich I, Gauch F, Weikert C. Nutritional Intake and Biomarker Status in Strict Raw Food Eaters. Nutrients. 2022;14(9). Epub 20220421. doi: 10.3390/nu14091725.

26. Chan Q, Stamler J, Brown IJ, Daviglus ML, Van Horn L, Dyer AR, et al. Relation of raw and cooked vegetable consumption to blood pressure: the INTERMAP Study. J Hum Hypertens. 2014;28(6):353-9. Epub 20131121. doi: 10.1038/jhh.2013.115.

27. Dordai L, Simedru D, Cadar O, Becze A. Simulated Gastrointestinal Digestion of Nutritive Raw Bars: Assessment of Nutrient Bioavailability. Foods. 2023;12(12). Epub 20230607. doi: 10.3390/foods12122300.

28. Fratianni A, D'Agostino A, Niro S, Bufano A, Paura B, Panfili G. Loss or Gain of Lipophilic Bioactive Compounds in Vegetables after Domestic Cooking? Effect of Steaming and Boiling. Foods. 2021;10(5). Epub 20210428. doi:10.3390/foods10050960.

29. Koebnick C, Strassner C, Hoffmann I, Leitzmann C. Consequences of a long-term raw food diet on body weight and menstruation: results of a questionnaire survey. Ann Nutr Metab. 1999;43(2):69-79. doi: 10.1159/000012770.

30. Kwanbunjan K, Koebnick C, Strassner C, Leitzmann C. Lifestyle and health aspects of raw food eaters. The Journal of Tropical Medicine and Parasitology. 2000;23(1):12-20.

31. Lee S, Choi Y, Jeong HS, Lee J, Sung J. Effect of different cooking methods on the content of vitamins and true retention in selected vegetables. Food Sci Biotechnol. 2018;27(2):333-42. Epub 20171212. doi:10.1007/s10068-017-0281-1.

32. Pahlavani N, Azizi-Soleiman F. The effects of a raw vegetarian diet from a clinical perspective; review of the available evidence. Clinical Nutrition Open Science. 2023;49:107-12. doi: 10.1016/j.nutos.2023.04.001.

33. Raba D-N, Iancu T, Bordean D-M, Adamov T, Popa V-M, Pîrvulescu LC. Pros and Cons of Raw Vegan Diet. Advanced Research in Life Sciences. 2019;3(1):46-51. doi: 10.2478/arls-2019-0010

34. Rodriguez-Ayala M, Banegas JR, Ortola R, Gorostidi M, Donat-Vargas C, Rodriguez-Artalejo F, et al. Cooking methods are associated with inflammatory factors, renal function, and other hormones and nutritional biomarkers in older adults. Sci Rep. 2022;12(1):16483. Epub 20221001. doi: 10.1038/s41598-022-19716-1.

35. Rodriguez-Ayala M, Sandoval-Insausti H, Bayan-Bravo A, Banegas JR, Donat-Vargas C, Ortola R, et al. Cooking Methods and Their Relationship with Anthropometrics and Cardiovascular Risk Factors among Older Spanish Adults. Nutrients. 2022;14(16). Epub 20220820. doi: 10.3390/nu14163426.

36. Rumm-Kreuter D, Demmel I. Comparison of vitamin losses in vegetables due to various cooking methods. Journal of Nutritional Science and Vitaminology. 1990;36(4-Supplement):S7-S15.

37. Yuan GF, Sun B, Yuan J, Wang QM. Effects of different cooking methods on health-promoting compounds of broccoli. J Zhejiang Univ Sci B. 2009;10(8):580-8. doi: 10.1631/jzus.B0920051.

Have a drink…

1. Afrose S, Sultana SSS, Zebsyn S, Binta Alam M, Huq AKO. Formulation of a detox health tonic diet for toxin elimination. International Journal of Life Sciences Research. 2023;11(2):58-62. doi: 10.5281/zenodo.8058436.

2. Almiron-Roig E, Chen Y, Drewnowski A. Liquid calories and the failure of satiety: how good is the evidence? Obes Rev. 2003;4(4):201-12. doi: 10.1046/j.1467-789x.2003.00112.x.

3. Ambulkar P, Hande P, Tambe B, Vaidya VG, Naik N, Agarwal R, et al. Efficacy and safety assessment of protein supplement - micronutrient fortification in promoting health and wellbeing in healthy adults - a randomized placebo-controlled trial. Transl Clin Pharmacol. 2023;31(1):13-27. Epub 20230302. doi:10.12793/tcp.2023.31.e1.

4. Brown MR, Klish WJ, Hollander J, Campbell MA, Forbes GB. A high protein, low calorie liquid diet in the treatment of very obese adolescents: long-term effect on lean body mass. The American journal of clinical nutrition. 1983;38(1):20-31.

5. Bryner RW, Ullrich IH, Sauers J, Donley D, Hornsby G, Kolar M, et al. Effects of resistance vs. aerobic training combined with an 800 calorie liquid diet on lean body mass and resting metabolic rate. J Am Coll Nutr. 1999;18(2):115-21.

6. Clark JE. Diets and Diet Therapy: Diet Supplements for Exercise. In: Ferranti P, Berry EM, Anderson JR, editors. Encyclopedia of Food Security and Sustainability. 2: Elsevier; 2019. p. 161-70.

7. Clark JE. Metabolism and nutrition: integration of concepts in a holistic approach to teaching metabolism. HAPS Educator. 2021;25(2):82-102. doi: 10.21692/haps.2021.026.

8. Cline JC. Nutritional aspects of detoxification in clinical practice. Altern Ther Health Med. 2015;21(3):54-63.

9. Garthe I, Maughan RJ. Athletes and Supplements: Prevalence and Perspectives. Int J Sport Nutr Exerc Metab. 2018;28(2):126-38. Epub 20180326. doi: 10.1123/ijsnem.2017-0429.

10. Graf S, Egert S, Heer M. Effects of whey protein supplements on metabolism: evidence from human intervention studies. Curr Opin Clin Nutr Metab Care. 2011;14(6):569-80. doi:10.1097/MCO.0b013e32834b89da.

11. Grundler F, Seralini GE, Mesnage R, Peynet V, Wilhelmi de Toledo F. Excretion of Heavy Metals and Glyphosate in Urine and Hair Before and After Long-Term Fasting in Humans. Front Nutr. 2021;8:708069. Epub 20210928. doi: 10.3389/fnut.2021.708069.

12. Harkness L. The history of enteral nutrition therapy: From raw eggs and nasal tubes to purified amino acids and early postoperative jejunal delivery. J Am Diet Assoc. 2002;102(3):399-404. doi: 10.1016/S0002-8223(02)90092-1.

13. Hodges RE, Minich DM. Modulation of Metabolic Detoxification Pathways Using Foods and Food-Derived Components: A Scientific Review with Clinical Application. J Nutr Metab. 2015;2015:760689. Epub 20150616. doi: 10.1155/2015/760689.

14. Hulmi JJ, Lockwood CM, Stout JR. Effect of protein/essential amino acids and resistance training on skeletal muscle hypertrophy: A case for whey protein. Nutr Metab (Lond). 2010;7:51. doi: 10.1186/1743-7075-7-51.

15. Klein AV, Kiat H. Detox diets for toxin elimination and weight management: a critical review of the evidence. J Hum Nutr Diet. 2015;28(6):675-86. Epub 20141218. doi: 10.1111/jhn.12286.

16. Maston G, Franklin J, Gibson AA, Manson E, Hocking S, Sainsbury A, et al. Attitudes and Approaches to Use of Meal Replacement Products among Healthcare Professionals in Management of Excess Weight. Behav Sci (Basel). 2020;10(9). Epub 20200907. doi: 10.3390/bs10090136

17. Mousa HA-L. Health effects of alkaline diet and water, reduction of digestive-tract bacterial load and earthing. Altern Ther Health Med. 2016;22(S1):24-33.

18. Noronha JC, Nishi SK, Braunstein CR, Khan TA, Blanco Mejia S, Kendall CWC, et al. The Effect of Liquid Meal Replacements on Cardiometabolic Risk Factors in Overweight/Obese Individuals With Type 2 Diabetes: A Systematic Review and Meta-analysis of Randomized Controlled Trials. Diabetes Care. 2019;42(5):767-76. Epub 20190328. doi: 10.2337/dc18-2270.

19. Patel V, Aggarwal K, Dhawan A, Singh B, Shah P, Sawhney A, et al. Protein supplementation: the double-edged sword. Proc (Bayl Univ Med Cent). 2024;37(1):118-26. Epub 20231220. doi: 10.1080/08998280.2023.2280417. PubMed PMID: 38174000; PubMed Central PMCID: PMCPMC10761008.

20. San Mauro Martin I, Barato VP, Rojo SS, Olivia SL, Vilar EG, Gudalewska P, et al. Are detox diets an effective strategy for obesity and oxidation management in short term? Journal of Negative & No Positive Results. 2017;2(9):399-409. doi: 10.19230/jonnpr.1585.

21. Savarino G, Corsello A, Corsello G. Macronutrient balance and micronutrient amounts through growth and development. Ital J Pediatr. 2021;47(1):109. Epub 20210508. doi: 10.1186/s13052-021-01061-0.

22. Sodano WL, Gristanti R, editors. The Physiology and Biochemistry of Biotransformation/Detoxification(The Phases of Detoxification)2010 Sep 16.

23. Sunardi D, Chandra DN, Medise BE, Manikam NRM, Friska D, Lestari W, et al. Health effects of alkaline, oxygenated, and demineralized water compared to mineral water among healthy population: a systematic review. Rev Environ Health. 2022. Epub 20221227. doi: 10.1515/reveh-2022-0057.

24. Tahreem A, Rakha A, Rabail R, Nazir A, Socol CT, Maerescu CM, et al. Fad Diets: Facts and Fiction. Front Nutr. 2022;9:960922. Epub 20220705. doi: 10.3389/fnut.2022.960922.

25. Tieken SM, Leidy HJ, Stull AJ, Mattes RD, Schuster RA, Campbell WW. Effects of solid versus liquid meal-replacement products of similar energy content on hunger, satiety, and appetite-regulating hormones in older adults. Horm Metab Res. 2007;39(5):389-94. doi: 10.1055/s-2007-976545.

26. Toni T, Alverdy J, Gershuni V. Re-examining chemically defined liquid diets through the lens of the microbiome. Nat Rev Gastroenterol Hepatol. 2021;18(12):903-11. Epub 20210930. doi: 10.1038/s41575-021-00519-0.

I am one with my food and my food is one with me…

1. Astrup A, Grunwald GK, Melanson EL, Saris WH, Hill JO. The role of low-fat diets in body weight control: a meta-analysis of ad libitum dietary intervention studies. International journal of obesity and related metabolic disorders : journal of the International Association for the Study of Obesity. 2000;24(12):1545-52.

2. Brown RE, Canning KL, Fung M, Jiandani D, Riddell MC, Macpherson AK, et al. Calorie Estimation in Adults Differing in Body Weight Class and Weight Loss Status. Med Sci Sports Exerc. 2016;48(3):521-6. doi: 10.1249/MSS.0000000000000796.

3. Chen J, Cade JE, Allman-Farinelli M. The Most Popular Smartphone Apps for Weight Loss: A Quality Assessment. JMIR mHealth and uHealth. 2015;3(4):e104. doi: 10.2196/mhealth.4334.

4. Cherpak CE. Mindful eating: A review of how the stress-digestion-mindfulness triad may modulate and improve gastrointestinal and digestive function. Integrative Medicine (Encinitas, Calif) 2019;18(4):48-53.

5. Clark JE. Metabolism and nutrition: integration of concepts in a holistic approach to teaching metabolism. HAPS Educator. 2021;25(2):82-102. doi: 10.21692/haps.2021.026.

6. Clark JE. A small switch in perspective: Comparing weight loss by nutrient balance versus caloric balance. Biol Sport. 2024. doi: 10.5114/biolsport.2024.133666.

7. Clark JE, Sirois E. Coercion versus self-selection when treating issues of overfatness: A narrative review. Health Educ J. 2023;82(5):475-86. Epub May 5, 2023. doi: 10.1177/00178969231171886.

8. Dunn C, Haubenreiser M, Johnson M, Nordby K, Aggarwal S, Myer S, et al. Mindfulness approaches and weight loss, weight maintenance, and weight regain. Current Obesity Reports. 2018;7:37-49. doi: 10.1007/s13679-018-0299-6.

9. Gudzune KA, Doshi RS, Mehta AK, Chaudhry ZW, Jacobs DK, Vakil RM, et al. Efficacy of commercial weight-loss programs: an updated systematic review. Ann Intern Med. 2015;162(7):501-12. doi: 10.7326/M14-2238.

10. Hall KD. What is the required energy deficit per unit weight loss? Int J Obes (Lond). 2008;32(3):573-6. doi:10.1038/sj.ijo.0803720.

11. Jia SS, Liu Q, Allman-Farinelli M, Partridge SR, Pratten A, Yates L, et al. The Use of Portion Control Plates to Promote Healthy Eating and Diet-Related Outcomes: A Scoping Review. Nutrients. 2022;14(4). Epub 20220220. doi: 10.3390/nu14040892.

12. Joachim-Celestin M, Rockwood NJ, Clarke C, Montgomery SB. Evaluating the Full Plate Living lifestyle intervention in low-income monolingual Latinas wit and without food insecurity. Women's Health. 2022;18:1-15. doi: 10.1177/17455057221091350.

13. Kelly RK, Calhoun J, Hanus A, Payne-Foster P, Stout R, Sherman BW. Increased dietary fiber is associated with weight loss among Full Plate Living program participants. Front Nutr. 2023;10:1110748. Epub 20230417. doi: 10.3389/fnut.2023.1110748.

14. Makovicky P, Makovicky P, Caja F, Rimarova K, Samasca G, Vannucci L. Celiac disease and gluten-free diet: past, present, and future. Gastroenterol Hepatol (N Y). 2020;13(1):1-7.

15. Nelson JB. Mindful Eating: The Art of Presence While You Eat. Diabetes Spectr. 2017;30(3):171-4. doi:10.2337/ds17-0015.

16. Tapper K. Mindful eating: what we know so far. Nutr Bull. 2022;47(2):168-85. Epub 20220510. doi:10.1111/nbu.12559.

17. Te Morenga LA, Levers MT, Williams SM, Brown RC, Mann J. Comparison of high protein and high fiber weight-loss diets in women with risk factors for the metabolic syndrome: a randomized trial. Nutr J. 2011;10:40.

18. Thomas DM, Martin CK, Lettieri S, Bredlau C, Kaiser K, Church T, et al. Can a weight loss of one pound a week be achieved with a 3500-kcal deficit? Commentary on a commonly accepted rule. Int J Obes (Lond). 2013;37(12):1611-3. doi: 10.1038/ijo.2013.51.

Curiouser and Curiouser…

Bland Diet

1. Robinson CH. Dietotherapy. The American Journal of Clinical Nutrition. 1954;2(3):206-10. doi: 10.1093/ajcn/2.3.206.

2. Cunningham E. Are low-residue diets still applicable. J Acad Nutr Diet. 2012;112(6). doi: 10.1016/j.jand.2012.04.005.

3. Weir SBS, Akhondi H. Bland Diet. Treasure Island, FL: StasPearls Publishing; 2023.

4. Vanhauwaert E, Matthys C, Verdonck L, De Preter V. Low-residue and low-fiber diets in gastrointestinal disease management. Adv Nutr. 2015;6(6):820-7. Epub 20151113. doi: 10.3945/an.115.009688.

5. Frankham P, Gosselin C, Cabanac M. Diet induced weight loss accelerates onset of negative alliesthesia in obese women. BMC Public Health. 2005;5:112. Epub 20051018. doi: 10.1186/1471-2458-5-112.

6. Dr. Peter D'Adamo's Blood Type Diet. www.dadamo.com visited 12.April.2024
7. University of Toronto. "Theory behind popular blood-type diet debunked." ScienceDaily. ScienceDaily, 15 January 2014. <www.sciencedaily.com/releases/2014/01/140115172246.htm
8. Cusack L, De Buck E, Compernolle V, Vandekerckhove P. Blood type diets lack supporting evidence: a systematic review. Am J Clin Nutr. 2013;98(1):99-104. Epub 20130522. doi: 10.3945/ajcn.113.058693.
9. Petroski W, Minich DM. Is There Such a Thing as "Anti-Nutrients"? A Narrative Review of Perceived Problematic Plant Compounds. Nutrients. 2020;12(10). Epub 20200924. doi: 10.3390/nu12102929.
10. Wang J, Garcia-Bailo B, Nielsen DE, El-Sohemy A. ABO genotype, 'blood-type' diet and cardiometabolic risk factors. PLoS One. 2014;9(1):e84749. Epub 20140115. doi: 10.1371/journal.pone.0084749.
11. Aljada B, Zohni A, El-Matary W. The Gluten-Free Diet for Celiac Disease and Beyond. Nutrients. 2021;13(11). Epub 20211109. doi: 10.3390/nu13113993.
12. Diez-Sampedro A, Olenick M, Maltseva T, Flowers M. A Gluten-Free Diet, Not an Appropriate Choice without a Medical Diagnosis. J Nutr Metab. 2019;2019:2438934. Epub 20190701. doi: 10.1155/2019/2438934.
13. Jones AL. The Gluten-Free Diet: Fad or Necessity? Diabetes Spectr. 2017;30(2):118-23. doi: 10.2337/ds16-0022.
14. Makovicky P, Makovicky P, Caja F, Rimarova K, Samasca G, Vannucci L. Celiac disease and gluten-free diet: past, present, and future. Gastroenterol Hepatol (N Y). 2020;13(1):1-7.
15. Melini V, Melini F. Gluten-Free Diet: Gaps and Needs for a Healthier Diet. Nutrients. 2019;11(1). Epub 20190115. doi: 10.3390/nu11010170.
16. Niland B, Cash BD. Health benefits and adverse effects of a gluten-free diet in non-celiac disease patients. Gastroenterol Hepatol (N Y). 2018;14(2):82-91.
17. Penagini F, Dilillo D, Meneghin F, Mameli C, Fabiano V, Zuccotti GV. Gluten-free diet in children: an approach to a nutritionally adequate and balanced diet. Nutrients. 2013;5(11):4553-65. Epub 20131118. doi:10.3390/nu5114553.
18. Posit Konigova M, Vnukova MS, Rehorkova P, Anders M, Ptacek R. The effectiveness of gluten-free dietary interventions: A systematic review. Front Psychol. 2023;14:1107022. doi: 10.3389/fpsyg.2023.1107022.
19. Reilly NR. The Gluten-Free Diet: Recognizing Fact, Fiction, and Fad. J Pediatr. 2016;175:206-10. Epub 20160513. doi: 10.1016/j.jpeds.2016.04.014.
20. Sabenca C, Ribeiro M, Sousa T, Poeta P, Bagulho AS, Igrejas G. Wheat/Gluten-Related Disorders and Gluten-Free Diet Misconceptions: A Review. Foods. 2021;10(8). Epub 20210730. doi: 10.3390/foods10081765.
21. Saturni L, Ferretti G, Bacchetti T. The Gluten-Free Diet: Safety and Nutritional Quality. Nutrients. 2010;2(1):16-34. doi: 10.3390/nu2010016.
22. Subhan FB, Chan CB. Review of Dietary Practices of the 21st Century: Facts and Fallacies. Can J Diabetes. 2016;40(4):348-54. doi: 10.1016/j.jcjd.2016.05.005.

A final take home message.

1. American College of Sports Medicine, American Dietetic Association AD, Dieticians of Canda Do. Nutrition and Athletic Performance. Med Sci Sports Exerc. 2009. doi: 10.1249/MSS.0b013e318190eb86. PubMed PMID: 19204578.
2. Byrne NM, Sainsbury A, King NA, Hills AP, Wood RE. Intermittent energy restriction improves weight loss efficiency in obese men: the MATADOR study. Int J Obes (Lond). 2018;42(2):129-38. doi: 10.1038/ijo 2017.206.
3. Chaix A, Zarrinpar A. The effects of time-restricted feeding on lipid metabolism and adiposity. Adipocyte. 2015;4(4):319-24. doi: 10.1080/21623945.2015.1025184.
4. Clark JE. A small switch in perspective: Comparing weight loss by nutrient balance versus caloric balance. Biol Sport. 2024. doi: 10.5114/biolsport.2024.133666.
5. Clark JE, Sirois E. Coercion versus self-selection when treating issues of overfatness: A narrative review. Health Educ J. 2023;82(5):475-86. Epub May 5, 2023. doi: 10.1177/00178969231171886.
6. Clark JE. Metabolism and nutrition: integration of concepts in a holistic approach to teaching metabolism. HAPS Educator. 2021;25(2):82-102. doi: 10.21692/haps.2021.026.
7. Clark JE. The impact of duration on effectiveness of exercise, the implication for periodization of training and goal setting for individuals who are overfat, a meta-analysis. Biol Sport. 2016;33(4):309-33. doi: 10.5604/20831862.1212974.
8. Da Poian AT, El-Bacha T, Luz MRMP. Nutrient utilization in humans: metabolism pathways. Nature Education. 2010;3(9):11.
9. Davis CS, Clarke RE, Coulter SN, Rounsefell KN, Walker RE, Rauch CE, et al. Intermittent energy restriction and weight loss: a systematic review. Eur J Clin Nutr. 2016;70(3):292-9. Epub 20151125. doi: 10.1038/ejcn.2015.195.
10. Di Francesco A, Di Germanio C, Brenier M, de Cabo R. A time to fast. Science. 2018;362:770-5.
11. Fern EB, Watzke H, Barclay DV, Roulin A, Drewnowski A. The nutrient balance concept: A new quality metric for composite meals and diets. PLoS One. 2015;10(7):e0130491. doi: 10.1371/journal.pone.0130491.
12. Freeland-Graves JH, Nitzke S, Academy of N, Dietetics. Position of the academy of nutrition and dietetics: total diet approach to healthy eating. J Acad Nutr Diet. 2013;113(2):307-17. doi: 10.1016/j.jand.2012.12.013.
13. Hall KD. Diet versus exercise in "the biggest loser" weight loss competition. Obesity. 2013;21(5):957-9. doi:10.1002/oby.20065.
14. Heikura IA, Stellingwerff T, Burke LM. Self-Reported Periodization of Nutrition in Elite Female and Male Runners and Race Walkers. Front Physiol. 2018;9:1732. Epub 20181203. doi: 10.3389/fphys.2018.01732.
15. Jeukendrup AE. Periodized Nutrition for Athletes. Sports Med. 2017;47(Suppl 1):51-63. doi: 10.1007/s40279-017-0694-2.

16. Jovanovski N, Jaeger T. Demystifying 'diet culture': Exploring the meaning of diet culture in online 'anti-diet' feminist, fat activist, and health professional communities. Women's Studies International Forum. 2022;90(January-February 2022):102558. doi: DOI: 10.1016/j.wsif.2021.102558.
17. Kerksick CM, Arent S, Schoenfeld BJ, Stout JR, Campbell B, Wilborn CD, et al. International society of sports nutrition position stand: nutrient timing. J Int Soc Sports Nutr. 2017;14:33. doi: 10.1186/s12970-017-0189-4.
18. Melzer K. Carbohydrate and fat utilization during rest and physical activity. E Spen Eur E J Clin Nutr Metab. 2011;6(2):e45-e52. doi: 10.1016/j.eclnm.2011.01.005.
19. National Institutes of Health, Office of Dietary Supplements (NIHODS). Nutrient Recommendations and Databases. https://ods.od.nih.gov/HealthInformation/nutrientrecommendations.aspx
20. Raiter N, Husnudinov R, Mazza K, Lamarche L. TikTok promotes diet culture and negative body image rhetoric: a content analysis. J Nutr Educ Behav. 2023;55(10):755-60. doi: 10.1016/j.neb.2023.08.001.
21. Rubin R. Backlash over meat dietary recommendations raises questions about corporate ties to nutrition scientists. JAMA. 2020;323(5):401-404. doi: 10.1001/jama.2019.21441.
22. Seimon RV, Roekenes JA, Zibellini J, Zhu B, Gibson AA, Hills AP, et al. Do intermittent diets provide physiological benefits over continuous diets for weight loss? A systematic review of clinical trials. Mol Cell Endocrinol. 2015;418 Pt 2:153-72. doi: 10.1016/j.mce.2015.09.014.
23. Tahreem A, Rakha A, Rabail R, Nazir A, Socol CT, Maerescu CM, et al. Fad Diets: Facts and Fiction. Front Nutr. 2022;9:960922. Epub 20220705. doi: 10.3389/fnut.2022.960922.
24. Tarnopolsky MA. Gender differences in metabolism; nutrition and supplements. Journal of science and medicine in sport / Sports Medicine Australia. 2000;3(3):287-98.
25. Zenone M, Ow N, Barbic S. TikTok and public health: a proposed research agenda. BMJ Glob Health. 2021;6(11). doi: 10.1136/bmjgh-2021-007648.